By Sheila Brook

All rights reserved, no part of this publication may be reproduced by any means, electronic, mechanical, or photocopying, documentary, film, or otherwise without prior permission of the publisher.

>Published by:
>Chipmunkapublishing
>PO Box 6872
>Brentwood
>Essex
>CM13 1ZT
>United Kingdom

http://www.chipmunkapublishing.com

Copyright © 2006 Sheila Brook

ISBN   978 1 84747 024 9

The development of this book was made possible by a grant from The Arts Council, London.

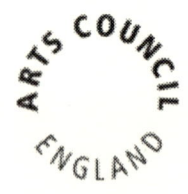

I DEDICATE THIS BOOK TO MY PARENTS

To my late father, whose constant anxiety and loneliness blended with courage, a buoyant and cheerful disposition in the face of much sorrow; and to commend my mother, about whom I knew so little, but whose illness and consequent 'life sentence' in Psychiatric Hospital deprived her of her home, her family and her freedom.

PREFACE

I felt constrained to write this book for several reasons. The world has changed so much during my lifetime that I wished to relate the memories of my childhood in the 1930s and during the War years. Initially I wanted to compare the innocence and simplicity of life during my childhood and the restrictions and scarcity of goods during the War, with the complexity and materialism of life today; to contrast the broken education the war produced with the wide facilities available in the twenty-first century.

Despite the deprivation caused by the War, and the repeated episodes of mental illness suffered by my mother, the recollections of contentment and comparative freedom during my childhood became clearer and more significant as I wrote. My mother's final psychiatric illness resulted in her spending the last fifty-three years of her life in Hospital. This meant my total separation from her for much of my childhood. As I wrote I appreciated more and more how hugely her illness must have affected my father's life and my own, as well as totally ending her own family and social life.

I then felt I would like to give some prominence to the many years my mother spent in Psychiatric Hospital, and to give recognition to my very private and isolated father, who rose above the many difficulties he had experienced in his life. I hope that my book will bring some value to my mother's life, that was so hidden, her experience so repressed, and that a greater understanding of mental illness will help to reduce the stigma still apparent today. Perhaps my story will also increase the awareness of the need for support for the relatives of those who are mentally ill.

Despite the war and the absence of my mother for most of my life, I have enjoyed revisiting my childhood and reliving many of the happy experiences. I believe that the divisions in my life caused by my mother's psychiatric illness have enabled me to retain many of my childhood memories in greater detail.

Chapter One

EARLY YEARS

I am a child of the thirties, born in the summer of 1931. I have many fragmented memories of my early years before the Second World War, as well as clear mental pictures of some other more major episodes in my early life. My mother had several severe nervous breakdowns during my childhood, and became seriously ill when I was eight years of age. The anxieties of the pre-war period may have affected her fragile nervous system, although I cannot remember any manic, aggressive or depressed behaviour in the period leading up to her final admission to psychiatric hospital a few months before the War began in September 1939. This was an unforgettable year for all who had lived through the early decades of the last century; the year that World War recurred after only twenty years of peace. The preceding months must have been a period of intense apprehension for everyone, especially for all who had survived the First World War, but even more so for people with a delicate nervous constitution such as my mother. What a brief period of peace my parents' generation had!

I am left with a collection of memories - but what are these memories made of? The flimsy bits and pieces that are recalled from the distant, or sometimes even the recent past seem to float across the screen of my mind of their own volition. Some are partially remembered as fragments of a dream. While my attention is focussed on them, other incidents are recalled, in the same way as one notices the details of a picture when scrutinising it carefully. Other events are retained in full detail as if I was looking at a photograph. Important events are completely, or almost completely, forgotten, although we are told they are as fully recorded in our minds as the unimportant flotsam that is so easily remembered. The episodes of my childhood that I can recall in detail make the years fall away, as the past is relived like a mental film show.

My only recollection of the day my mother was once again admitted to a Mental Hospital in the summer of 1939 is of my father waking me up early one morning. As I roused from my sleep he gently shook me on the shoulder and told me very quietly to get dressed quickly. There was no sign of my mother as we left the house before breakfast. I didn't question what was happening as we walked rapidly along the street. My father knocked on the door of a neighbour's house and a few hurried words were exchanged with a lady I knew. I was left in her care and I surmised that she was going to look after me until it was time for school. I don't recollect my father explaining to me why my mother was not around and I never knew what crisis may have occurred after I had gone to bed the previous night. Had my mother left the house and been taken to hospital? Was she still at home when I was taken to the neighbour's house?

I will never know what happened. I can't remember whether my mother had behaved strangely, appeared unwell or over-excited the previous day and I certainly had no idea that when I saw her again she would be a grandmother! I had no opportunity to say 'good-bye' to her. I had no idea of the many changes that were about to occur in our family, but the deserted early morning streets are easily recalled and seemed to bear down on me with a vague sense of uncertainty and gloom as I hurried along holding my father's hand. After this sudden separation my mother was rarely spoken of, and I did not see her again for over twenty years. The brief periods of normal family life I had experienced with both my parents would not occur again.

Recollections of the first part of that day are hazy, but I clearly remember sitting cross-legged on the floor in my School Hall during Assembly later that morning – I needed to blow my nose. I had left home in some bewilderment, in such a rush, and without a handkerchief. I don't think that I had been crying, as I had not understood what had happened, but I whispered to my classmate, David, who was sitting next to me, asking him if I could borrow his handkerchief to blow my nose. What a strange insignificant detail to be recalled from the storehouse of my mind!

When I next saw my mother early in 1960 she had responded well to the new anti-psychotic drugs that had been developed after the War. She was then in her sixties and I was a married woman with two children. I didn't recognise her when we met in the gardens of the Hospital in which she had been a patient for over twenty years, but we greeted each other quite warmly, although perhaps a little hesitantly. She had been told that 'Sheila' was coming to see her but she couldn't accept that I was her daughter. On subsequent visits she was unable to recall any incidents of my childhood when she was at home and well, or acknowledge that the Aunt and Uncle I referred to in our conversations were her own sister and brother-in-law. Perhaps the courses of electro-convulsive therapy she had been given during her long years in hospital had wiped much of her previous life from her memory. I soon began to visit her regularly, together with my father and my family. She chatted with us all, but insisted that my sons were not her grandsons and I was not her daughter. She asserted that she had had two daughters and 'they' had taken them both away from her. In a sense this was true.

My mother was thirty-five and my father was two years older when I arrived (unexpectedly?) on the scene in the summer of 1931. By that time my parents had been married for eleven years and their first daughter had been born nine years previously. Years had passed by before I knew I had had a sister who died. I therefore grew up as an only child, as this unknown sister had died many years before I was born. Peggy was never mentioned in conversation, but I clearly remember how I first heard about her.

I was about ten years old, or maybe even older, when I learned this information while putting a spoonful of tea into the teapot one day. We had an old, tarnished, silver spoon in our tea caddy, engraved with the name 'Peggy' in elaborate letters on the handle, and I asked my father who 'Peggy' was. He briefly told me that the spoon had been a christening gift for my sister who had been born a long time before me, but that she had had fits and had died while still a baby. I didn't know what 'fits' meant, but it sounded nasty, as my father seemed ill at ease and reluctant to say any more about her; I asked no further questions. I was very much older when I heard the term epilepsy used, and learned that Peggy had been brain-damaged at birth.

She was never spoken of again - until I talked to my mother about her fifty years later, and she said that Peggy had been born blind, deaf and suffered from epilepsy. My mother told me that Peggy had died when she was about eighteen months old. My mother said that she had not attended her funeral, but she had seen her baby daughter carried out of the house in a little box. I will never know whether all the details of this information are true, but it would seem that my parents buried their unspoken grief with their daughter and never wished to speak of her again. Poor, forgotten Peggy!

My parents were living in a semi-detached house in the developing suburb of Osterley, on the outskirts of London when I was born. I can just remember the wide, busy highway at the top end of our road, and in later years I learned that this was the Great West Road - now the A4. At the time I lived in the area it was not a busy, congested thoroughfare, but Osterley is now absorbed into Greater London and on the flight path for Heathrow. I have almost no memory of my early years in the house of my birth. I can visualise nothing of the inside of the house that for some periods was my home during the first four years of my life, although I am sure that an enamel-topped, black-edged table was in daily use in the kitchen, as indeed it continued to be for many decades in our next home. I have no memories of playing with toys, being bathed, read to, or put to bed at night and can recall no memories of being with my mother.

Mental pictures of my early childhood are almost non-existent, with the faint exception of struggling to get a child's metal 'pedal car' to move in the right direction, or even to move at all, as I pushed furiously on the pedals, trying to 'drive' up our sideway in the same way that my father drove his car into the garage each evening. I guess that the old-fashioned, red painted, pedal car would only run - even then reluctantly - on concrete or on paving stones. I can bring back the sense of frustration after the passage of seventy years, and think this must be my earliest memory. This little incident is associated with the outside of the house, either in our driveway or along the pavement. I recall nothing of being indoors or playing in the garden.

At the bottom of our road was a high brick wall, which marked the boundary of the stately home of Lord Jersey. Only five years after my family moved from Osterley the first organised training of the Home Guard was undertaken in the grounds of Osterley House during the summer of 1940. The House and Gardens now belong to the National Trust and are open to the public, but in the nineteen thirties the Estate was still privately owned, and the Grounds were opened to the local community on one day each year. The other side of the high brick wall that surrounded the Estate was unknown territory to me as a toddler, but I wonder whether my parents visited the Gardens, or if I was ever pushed around the paths in my 'bassinet' (as a pram was called in those days) on 'Open Day'. My parents may not even have known who owned Osterley House. I fear they had other concerns as my mother had recurring episodes of mental illness. I have returned to Osterley in recent years, and looked at the outside of the house where I was born in Penwerris Avenue, but nothing about the facade seemed in any way familiar.

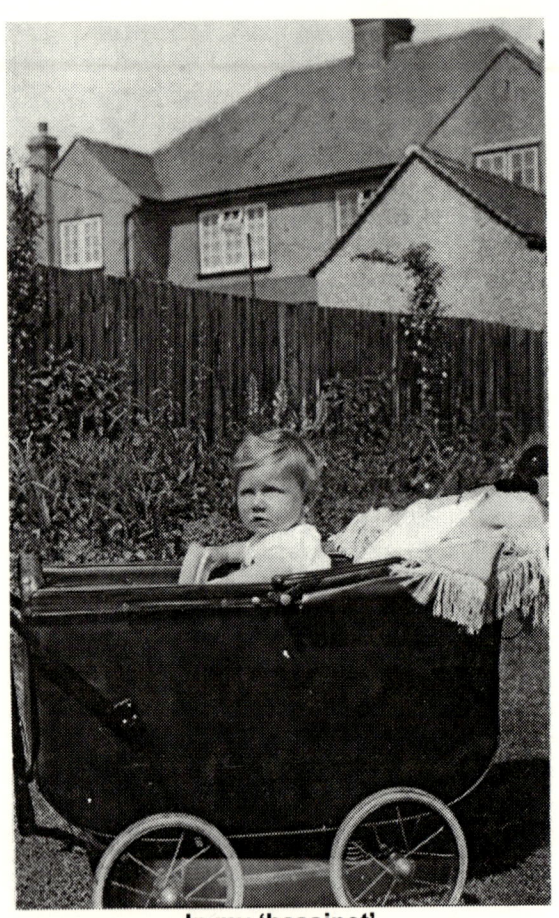

In my 'bassinet'.

I don't know when I first realised that my mother was not well, or if I was ever aware of anything abnormal in her behaviour. I have no memory of when I first heard the term 'nervous breakdown', but I understand that my mother became ill when I was still very young. I was not much more than a toddler and have no memory of the time I first stayed with my Aunt and Uncle Connell. Old photographs are my only evidence. I was too young to be aware that the sudden change in my circumstances was unusual. There is, I suppose, the possibility that I was at risk and had to be removed from home if a crisis occurred.

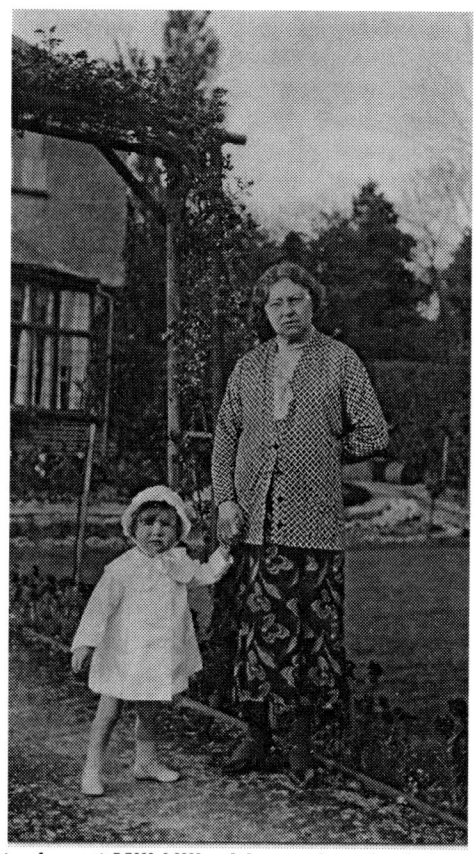

Staying at Mill Hill with my Auntie Connell

I do remember living with another Aunt and Uncle some time later, and recall my Auntie Ada undoing the hard round buttons on my little black patent-leather shoes with the aid of a buttonhook. I also needed assistance with the rows of tiny buttons down the outside of the 'leggings' small children wore when going out in those days, so I realise that even then I was still not much more than a toddler. I vaguely recollect being very ill with one of the dangerous childhood infectious diseases while living with this Aunt and Uncle. These were serious and sometimes life-threatening conditions, and I can recall my Aunt's and my Uncle Bert's, anxiety and concern. The bedroom doorway was covered with a white sheet, and an electric light glowed dimly throughout the night. There were 'comings and goings' in and out of the bedroom where I lay in a large, brass-knobbed double bed. A dark-clothed, large, unknown male figure looked down at me and I overheard solemn, whispered voices. There were further visits from the heavily built, solemn adult, presumably the doctor, who placed his large black hat on the bed while he examined me. I was aware of my Aunt's worried demeanour and I believe that I was seriously ill for a while, but I have never known from what I had suffered. My Aunt was responsible for me while my mother was ill; she and my Uncle had no children of their own. She had no experience of dealing with childhood illnesses and this may have added to her anxiety.

I did not understand that my mother was in Hospital when living with these relations. I would certainly not have understood the significance of the terms 'Mental Home', 'Asylum', or 'Mental Hospital' either and probably did not even know what the word 'Hospital' meant. The expression 'Psychiatric Hospital' would not have been used in those days.

I have a faint memory of hearing raised voices as I played in the hallway of some friends my parents often visited. When I was much older my father told me that there were occasional rather heated political discussions while drinking tea (or sipping sherry) and chatting with these friends. I had no understanding of the reason of the arguments, or even whether they were arguments, but I can remember the raised voices. It is strange that this indistinct memory has enabled me to recall more about the interior of Dr. and Mrs. Carr's house than I can remember about my own first home. I also remember walking home one evening, hand in hand with my father and Dr. Carr. Were the two gentlemen taking me home because my mother had become over-excited and 'flipped'? Had she become aggressive with their politically minded friends, or with my father? Was Mrs. Carr looking after her? Had my mother become ill again, and was she possibly on her way to Hospital? I don't know, but I sense that I was being removed from some minor (or major) crisis. As far as I am aware, my father never held strong, dogmatic political views but it would seem that these friends were arousing their - or perhaps just my mother's - political fervour, and a clash of opinions had resulted in an altercation. The heightened voices were imprinted on my memory, together with the silent walk home with my father and his friend in the dusk.

Many, many years later my cousin Daphne told me that my mother apparently also had heated political discussions with my Uncle Jack, Daphne's father. I find it difficult to believe that she could have held such strong political opinions, but maybe this was one way in which her mental instability was expressed. My cousin also revealed to me that her mother had told her that I was sometimes shut up in the cupboard under the stairs, and that my mother was sometimes not well enough to look after me properly. I have no recollection of any such frightening occurrences. I sometimes stayed with my Auntie Lily and Uncle Jack for short periods; I didn't understand or wonder why I had these sudden extended 'holidays' alone, and not in the company of my parents.

They were holidays with a difference, and became temporary second 'homes' for me. After my mother died in 1992 at the great age of ninety-six, I learned from an interview with her Psychiatric Consultant that her records indicated that she had had several nervous breakdowns, with periods in Hospital when I was young, which at last explained to me the reason for these unexpected 'holidays'. Although my father told me that my mother had initially been diagnosed as suffering from mania, I sometimes wonder whether she developed post-natal depression after my birth. She may never have got over the loss of her first daughter. I understand that the shock of discovering Peggy's disability, the stress of caring for her before her sudden death precipitated a period of deep depression after Peggy died. This may have seriously affected my mother's mental health, or may have made her unduly fearful during her second (unplanned, I am sure) pregnancy. There was little understanding of mental illness at that time; post-natal depression had not been recognised. Even if the cause of, or possible emotional reason for, my mother's 'life-sentence' was known, there was little treatment available until the early 1950s. People were often shut away and sometimes abandoned by their families, who felt there was no hope of recovery from a severe mental illness.

I have a little snippet of memory that may relate to the development of my mother's next mental illness in 1935. Many years later my father told me that she had had some dispute with the neighbours, and I recalled a faint memory of once hearing raised voices and shouting from our kitchen door as I played in our driveway. I have no other recollections of my mother being over-excited, but it was after this remembered incident of loud voices over the fence that divided the two houses that I found myself once again suddenly separated from both my parents, and I never returned to our home in Osterley. This time I was not staying with relatives for an unexpected 'holiday', but with people I had not met before, and with whom I lived for some months.

I presume my father found this refuge or temporary 'home' for me, and my next clear memory is of living in a Victorian villa in West Ealing with two people whom I came to know as Miss Skinner and her brother. This time I understood that my mother was in hospital. My father took me to visit her one Sunday afternoon, and we walked up a driveway towards some 'institutional-looking' building, which I believe was the outside of St. Bernard's Hospital in Southall. A nurse brought my mother outside and I met with her briefly in the grounds of the Hospital. I can only remember standing in the Drive leading up to the Hospital, and can visualise the nurse in her white uniform, but have no recollection of how my mother responded to seeing me, or of my emotions at seeing her after an absence of some time.

I have discovered that St. Bernard's Hospital was originally a 'model county lunatic asylum, incorporating many unique Victorian purpose-built features'. It is now a museum, 'telling the story of its first two humane governors and its subsequent history, which is a microcosm of changes in treating the mentally ill and handicapped'. This description is given in a brochure published by Ealing Borough Council, where St. Bernard's Hospital Museum is now listed as a tourist attraction! At least treatment was kinder than in the eighteenth century when the mentally ill were considered to be a 'tourist attraction', and the public paid money to come to Bedlam (Bethlem Hospital in London) and watch the poor patients being cruelly and heartlessly treated. St. Bernard's Hospital Museum gives some idea of what life might have been like for my mother and other mentally ill people before the arrival of modern treatment. Many other mental institutions were, no doubt, less enlightened in those days and my mother could have endured far bleaker, harsher conditions if she had been in a different part of the country. The Women's Ward of an Asylum may not have been considered a suitable place to take a young child into in the 1930s and could account for my very faint recollection of only the outside of the Hospital. Indeed, it was still deemed unsuitable for me to go into her Ward in 1960, when as an adult I first saw my mother again in the grounds of Shenley Hospital in Hertfordshire.

I remember a number of things connected with the house I lived in while my mother was in St. Bernard's Hospital, but my clearest memories are of the motherliness and kindness of Miss Skinner herself and of her brother's twinkling eyes and sense of humour. He often teased me. I nicknamed him 'Teaser' (although his sister probably suggested this name and I just adopted it. I don't think I was cheeky enough to have called him 'Teaser' of my own volition!) Both he and his sister seemed quite old to me, although I could not have had a very accurate idea of age when I was barely four years old myself. I have little visual memory of the inside of their house, apart from a vague recollection of the front reception room (called the parlour) and I only remember going into this room on one very special occasion. I had a washstand with a large jug and bowl in my bedroom, but have no idea what my bedroom was like, or if there was a bathroom in the house.

My clearest memory is of a large kind of conservatory, which extended across the whole of the back of the house. It was glass-roofed and supported by thin metal pillars. It didn't seem like a conservatory, as one understands the word nowadays. It was a large, glass-covered canopy and was a much-used living space in the summer months that was completely open to the garden along the outer side. An 'outside' lavatory under the glass roofed, canopied extension made a visit to the 'little house' a real convenience!

There was a large, frequently scrubbed, plain wooden table in the middle of the conservatory, on which food was prepared, pastry made, or the ironing done, where I sat and watched Miss Skinner at her work, or looked through the old-fashioned books she produced for me. I cannot recall playing with any toys. We ate at this table too and it was the hub of the house as far as I was concerned. This 'garden room' was much more used, lived in and worked in than the little kitchen or scullery that it adjoined and I do not recall eating in a dining room. I spent quite a lot of time sitting at the table, feeling a little bored as I turned the pages of the books I could not yet read, pausing to look at the occasional pictures I found. One of the books was a copy of Don Quixote and I don't quite know why I remember this, but the title has stuck in my mind. Maybe it had pictures in it, but I found it very uninteresting. I doubt whether I recognised the feeling as boredom at the time, as I think I was an uncomplaining child and accepted without comment what life meted out.

Miss Skinner's garden was my main diversion and play area although it contained nothing of specific interest for children. It was an old-fashioned town garden, without any lawn, but with several large square beds surrounded by little brick paths. These large beds were full of roses and other flowers, vegetables and soft-fruit bushes - currants, raspberries and gooseberries. I clearly remember all these fruits and can even recall peeping under the branches of the bushes to search for a ripe, reddish-skinned, hairy gooseberry, and staining my fingers on some luscious, juicy raspberries I found there. No wonder I enjoyed wandering down the little pathways! They were bordered with low wavy-edged, red tiles and I passed many hours contentedly on my own in this tranquil garden.

'Teaser' was either retired, out of work, or on some kind of shift work, as he was often around during the daytime. The Skinners had a friendly, shaggy dog, named 'Snip', and 'Teaser' and I, together with the dog, often went for walks into nearby Walpole Park. We paused by the little round goldfish pond near the entrance, leaning on the black, ornamental iron railings that surrounded the pond, waiting for the fish to appear from beneath the lily pads that almost covered the surface of the water. It was a very large park, with a stream, a rock garden and many paths to stroll along and a spacious area of grass for children to play on. I don't remember playing ball with 'Teaser', but we paid regular visits to what appeared to me to be an impressive aviary tucked away in a corner, where a variety of tropical birds - budgerigars, canaries, macaws and two vividly coloured parrots - sat on their perches. The parrots took most of my attention and interest. 'Teaser' and I spent a long time watching them and encouraging them to talk. One parrot was usually silent but we had little difficulty in coaxing his mate to squawk "Hello" and "Pretty Polly" to us. I thought 'Polly' was a wonderful creature with her brilliantly coloured, exotic feathers.

I enjoyed all these amenities in Walpole Park in the mid-1930s and have clear and happy memories of our regular walks with 'Snip'. I think that 'Teaser' enjoyed our outings too. Walpole Park was little changed when I last visited it. The round pond was still near the entrance, with its railings as I remembered them from so long ago, but looking a little dilapidated and I saw no goldfish swimming in its murky water. My father told me many years ago that he and my mother used to play tennis with friends on the tennis courts in Lammas Park at the far end of Walpole Park before I was born. I have an old photo of my parents amongst a group of tennis players, holding their heavy, wooden-framed racquets as they sat in deck chairs after a game. The men are wearing their white 'flannels' and most have cigarettes between their lips. The ladies look charming with their rather lengthy white dresses and white bandeaux around the Eton crop hairstyles so popular in the nineteen-twenties. I am glad my parents had some happy times before my mother became so ill.

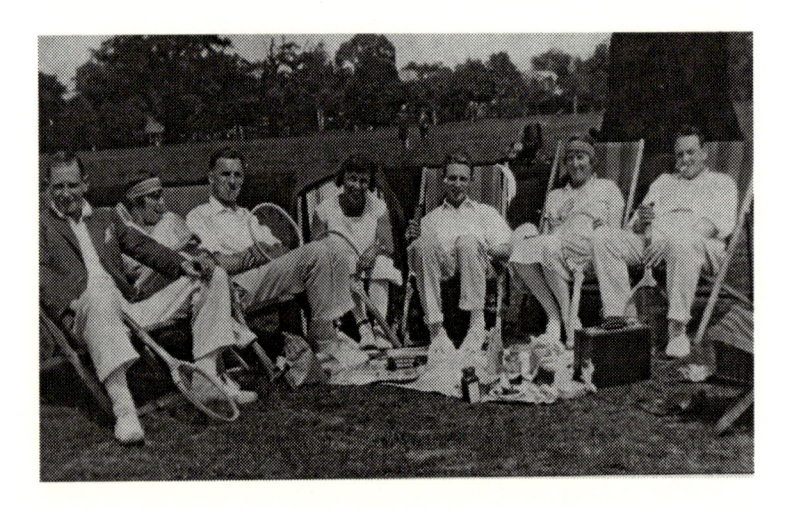

After a game of tennis in the park

My mother was not spoken about while I was living with Miss Skinner. Even at that age I think I sensed that inquiries would be inappropriate - but perhaps I should have asked questions. Maybe my father was waiting for these questions from me, but I sensed that nobody wanted to talk about her at all. Mental illness was considered to be such a shameful condition in those days; one that close relatives found hard to come to terms with and received little, if any, understanding from others. Yet they needed so much support. Is society much more compassionate and comprehending today? I am not sure. This uncomfortable, embarrassed, shameful feeling about mental illness transferred itself to me when I was a child.

I don't know what treatment my mother may have received in St. Bernard's Hospital. I know she had ECT a number of times during her lifetime and she may have had the drug lithium. There was little other treatment available before the post-war development of tranquillisers, anti-depressants and anti-psychotic medication. Something must have helped her because after some months my father brought my mother to see me at Miss Skinner's home. She may have been on a brief 'home' visit', or had possibly been discharged from Hospital; I can only remember feeling somewhat uncomfortable as we met together in Miss Skinner's front parlour after what seemed like a long period of separation. My mother had apparently made a reasonable recovery, but I can remember a sense of uneasiness between both my parents and myself, of not knowing how to behave or quite what to say. There were certainly no warm embraces.

Long afterwards my father told me that it was thought that it would be better for my mother to move to a different house when she came out of Hospital and to live in a new locality that would not evoke unhappy memories of her old home that might disturb her. A completely new environment could be the means of stabilising her mental health. Although I have searched my memory for incidents of irrationality, hysterical laughter or undue excitement in those early years, I can remember nothing of real significance apart from the two occasions of raised voices - the row with a neighbour and the heated political argument with friends. I have no recollection of the excited political discussions with my Uncle Jack. These may have had nothing to do with her mental state. Holding or expressing strong views is not necessarily a sign of mental instability! It is quite probable that other incidents occurred of which I was either unaware, or whose memory is buried too deeply for me to recall.

My father used the term mania to describe my mother's illness. None of the recognised symptoms of manic depression - elation, euphoria, delusions, over-self-confidence are compatible with any of my faint memories of her. I cannot recall any incoherent speech or incessant activity - but neither can I recall many of her actions or conversations with me when I was a small child. My father has told me that she had suffered very severely in the epidemic (or pandemic) of influenza towards the end of World War One and he felt that her personality had changed after her recovery. Although this may not have been relevant to her subsequent history, my father thought it was related. Lack of proper diagnosis or effective treatment in those days may have led to a deep inner frustration and a worsening of her symptoms, the subsequent development of schizophrenia and the severe mental illness she suffered for the rest of her life.

Mental Hospitals were comfortless institutions (but often in peaceful, but isolated, surroundings), with locked Wards, padded rooms for violent patients, little in the way of curative or alleviating treatment and in some case not much warmth or kindness. Strength, firm control and restraint when necessary, were essential requirements for nursing staff. A cigarette was often given to calm patients, almost as a form of medication, even up until the end of the 1980s'! The depressed or withdrawn would often become even more so, as 'talking' was not yet recognised as a helpful therapy. Recovery must have been considered less of a possibility than a lifetime's residence in an institution. Many patients were completely forsaken by their relatives, who could not stand the strain or the stigma caused by the many more or less untreatable forms of mental illness. Life was bleak for patient and relatives alike.

Chapter Two

ON THE MOVE

However, my mother did recover and my father was hopeful that a completely new start would bring happiness and stability to their (and my) lives. I was still living with Miss Skinner when my parents arrived one day to take me off in my father's Baby Austin Seven car to look at a new house on a small development of modern houses at Kenton, near Harrow, in Middlesex (now part of Greater London).

I clearly remember being shown round this newly built, bright, empty house by the estate agent, a rather stout gentleman. The external walls of the group of about two-dozen houses had a white rendered finish. This whiteness was very distinctive and memorable to me. The smooth 'Snowcemmed' finish was different from all the pebble-dashed walls I had seen on the houses in Osterley, or the mellow brick walls of the old terraced houses in Miss Skinner's area of West Ealing. The attractive subtle green tiles on the roofs were in great contrast to the other houses in the neighbourhood and were a suggestion of what I later learned was the Modernist style of architecture in the thirties. The interior of the house also made a strong impression on me, possibly because it was the first totally empty house I had ever entered, and the bare floorboards made a loud noise as I walked around the rooms and up the uncarpeted wooden staircase. The house agent took us along the road to show my parents how near we would be to the parade of local shops, and I overheard him tell them that the Infants' School was a little way up the road by the shops. This was no doubt an important point to emphasise, as I would soon be starting school.

This new house was the only one that I went in, although my father may have viewed other properties before taking my mother and me to see the one he favoured. The district must have seemed eminently suitable to him. It was a newly developing suburb, well away from any major highway as in Osterley. The style of the house was very different from the one we had been living in, with its modern architecture and somewhat avant-garde interior and so would not provoke unhappy memories for my mother. Although I lived in this house for many, many years, through the rest of my childhood and teenage years, and until long after I was married, I am sure that the initial impressions were fixed in my memory during that first visit with the house agent. It was the first really 'modern' house I had seen, with what I subsequently learned were called 'sun-trap' windows. Every room had large windows, with the windows of the front reception room curving round towards the porch. These Crittall window frames were made of galvanized iron and were a modern innovation of the thirties. The metal frames would do away for ever with the risk of rotting wooden window frames - but the designers had not recognised that rust would soon develop from condensation collecting along the thin edges of each frame during the winter months. That, however, is a much later memory, and knowledge that was acquired after many years' experience of helping to mop up pools of water on the window ledges during the cold winters of the War, then drying off the metal frames with a cloth, to try and retard the development of rust. One did not contemplate repainting in wartime, and nobody had begun to think of rust-resistant, low-maintenance UPVC window and doorframes then!

The lightness of the interior of the house impressed me. The clear glass doors dividing the two reception rooms made the entire living area appear bright and spacious. There were no picture rails; the walls were finished in light, textured paper, with a decorative frieze that was stepped in an up-to-date zigzag style in the corners, and an added floral motif. The light-fittings in the reception rooms were very contemporary in style, with chrome ceiling fittings supporting upturned, opaque, pale-green, shallow glass bowls. There were smart, triangular-shaped glass wall lights and pastel-colored tiled fire surrounds, with no old-fashioned wooden over mantels. I am sure I didn't appreciate any of the details of this Art Deco style at the time, but the lightness and the soft colors are very early memories. The skirting boards were shaped in what was then a modern zigzag style, and all the interior woodwork was painted in a light creamy yellow with a textured finish.

I saw the house again towards the end of the century; it has stood the test of time. The exterior still looks smart and well maintained, although a large extension has completely changed the interior character. Our old back garden was almost unrecognisable. It appeared much shorter because of the extension and the large cherry tree at the bottom of the garden had been replaced with a large outbuilding. All the fruit trees I remembered from my childhood had gone and the garden looked sad and uncared for.

We moved to Kenton in the summer of 1935, but I remember nothing of the removal, and believe that I remained with Miss Skinner until after my parents had settled in to their new home, hoping for an untroubled future. My earliest mental picture of our life at Kenton is of my father digging over the expanse of rough earth at the back of the house. He was levelling the ground so that grass seed could be sown to form a lawn before the winter weather came along. The following year three rustic arches were placed in position; one was erected halfway down the garden at the end of the path that ran alongside our garage and two others were fixed into the earth to the right and left of the lower end of the lawn. My parents planted a number of fruit trees - a cherry at the bottom of the garden, with a Bramley apple tree at each side and two plum trees nearer the house.

The fruit from these trees supplied us with an abundance of plums and apples during the War and for many years after. I have very strong memories of the bottling process that was carried out each summer during my youth and early adulthood. Large old jam jars were filled to the brim with Victoria and golden plums and placed on an asbestos mat in the oven. The gas was turned down very low and the fruit was slowly heated until it looked cooked, when the jars of plums were taken from the oven one at a time. Each one was filled to the brim with boiling water to exclude all the air, quickly capped with a metal lid and sealed with a clip. The following day we tested the strength of the vacuum seal by removing the clip and lifting each jar carefully by its metal lid. If the lid stayed on we knew that the seal was strong and the contents were airtight. The jars of delicious fruit were then ranged along a shelf in the larder with great satisfaction and used during the winter. A jar was taken down almost every week to provide a dish of stewed plums or a plum pie as a treat after our Sunday dinner.

The apples were wrapped in newspaper and stored in boxes in the garage. They were examined from time to time to check that they were keeping well. Some inevitably rotted as the winter months passed by, but in the main they kept us well supplied with fruit for the baked apples, apple pies and tarts made during the War by my father's housekeeper. The fruit from these trees was much appreciated in the years of shortage during and after the War.

As the white-heart cherry tree matured it also produced a good crop of large sweet cherries. The birds shared these; they always seemed to know just when the fruit was at its best. They sometimes got to the crop before my father had had the opportunity of propping his ladder up against the tree and picking the luscious, pink-tinged cherries. In later years our lawn was liberally sprinkled with the discarded cherrystones every summer after the birds had eaten more than their fair share of the crop. The cherry tree grew quickly and eventually became a very large specimen that dominated the bottom of our garden – the new, large, man-made structure now occupies that position!

I cannot be certain exactly when the fruit trees were planted, or how quickly the garden developed, but the seeding of the lawn and the arrival of the arches and trees occurred very soon after we moved in. I can vaguely remember my mother helping my father in all this work. Rustic arches and young trees can be seen in all the photos that were taken in the garden before my mother became very seriously ill again four years later. She only had four short years in which to enjoy her new home and garden. Sadly, she had little opportunity to benefit - literally - from the fruits of her labours.

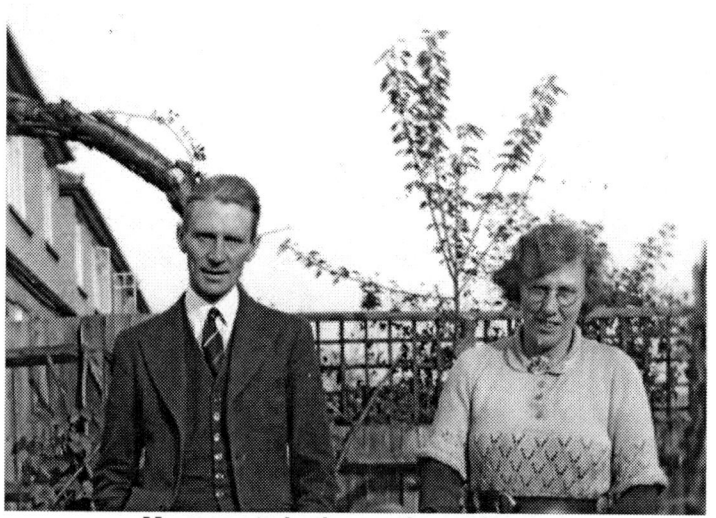

My parents in the garden at Kenton

My large bedroom at the back of the house overlooked the garden. It faced east and was very bright and sunny in the mornings. Two built-in cupboards at either end of one wall were painted with a textured light, pastel-colored effect. A two-kilowatt electric fire with a pale green tiled surround was a neat fixture on the wall opposite my bed. There was no need for a fireplace in my bedroom and consequently there was no chimneybreast. When Christmas time came I wondered how Father Christmas could deliver my presents without a chimney to climb down and my parents made up the story that he came through the bedroom window in an airplane to bring me my gifts. This idea frightened the life out of me and I had to be rescued from my fear by having the magic of Father Christmas dispelled with the truth. I sometimes wonder what story is fabricated for children who live in present-day homes with no fireplaces or chimneys at all!

My parents slept in the main front bedroom, which had a small tiled fireplace and a chimneybreast, although I never saw a fire in the grate. There was a third, small bedroom above the hall. The bathroom had the modern convenience of a hot towel rail, with water heated by the boiler in the kitchen below coming up to the hot-water tank in the airing cupboard in the bathroom and thence to the towel rail. This gave us a very cosy bathroom and kept the towels dry and warm – quite a luxury in those days.

Modern (for the period) units were fitted along one side of the kitchen, with cupboards and drawers of various sizes and an extra work surface provided by a large flap that could be dropped down when necessary. The far end of the kitchen had a red-tiled floor and just inside the back door was a large, deep, traditional porcelain sink with an enamel draining board and built-in cupboards beneath. A wooden plate rack was fitted on the wall above the sink. I have never lived in a house without a plate rack in my kitchen. It's the nearest I have been to owning a dishwasher! The small old-fashioned gas stove had no temperature control; the gas tap was gently turned up or down to get more or less heat. A clothes boiler was in a corner beside the gas stove and a large hand wringer with wooden rollers was kept in the back garden and covered over when not in use.

There was room for a table (the enamel-topped one from our old house) to prepare food on and we always ate our breakfast here after the War started. I cannot remember eating a meal at the kitchen table when my mother was at home; I think we always sat at the dining table. Our kitchen table always seemed old-fashioned to me, but it was wonderfully cool and smooth for rolling out pastry and the enamel was very easy to keep clean and hygienic. The solid fuel boiler provided all the hot water for the household and kept the kitchen warm and cosy during the winter. The larder was situated on the south side of the house, making it difficult to keep food fresh in the summer. A small window covered with wire mesh on the outside wall allowed fresh air to circulate. A large, tiled, deep shelf in the larder helped to keep food reasonably cool, although during hot weather nothing would have been anywhere near the +4 degrees C required nowadays. This completed our nineteen-thirties kitchen. It must have seemed very modern and streamlined at the time.

Very few people had a refrigerator before the nineteen-fifties and as I grew older I soon became familiar with the schemes devised to keep food fresh in the summer. We stood the glass bottles of milk in a pan of cold water and draped a muslin cloth over the tops of the bottles with its edges dipping into the water. Our Sunday joint was thoroughly wiped over with a cloth wrung out in vinegar before being roasted, in order to kill any 'nasties' that had developed on it overnight. I doubt whether my mother, or our housekeeper a few years later, had ever heard of the word 'bacteria' and food sometimes spoiled or went 'off' in hot weather. The milk would go sour, the cheese turned hard and waxy, the bacon became tough, discolored and greasy, the butter was soft and oily, and green vegetables or lettuce became limp. I am sure the meat was sometimes tainted, but we cooked it well; we survived, and apart from an occasional stomach upset, there were very few gastric infections in the family.

The front reception room was always called the dining room, but it was our main living room. The square oak dining table had carved bulbous legs and deep grooves were carved in the tabletop, which could be extended by pulling out both ends. Four heavy dining chairs had the same style of carved legs. The leatherbacks and seats were fixed with brass studs around all the edges. Oak stretcher bars connected the legs of each item of furniture and gave added strength. This 'Jacobethan' style was popular in the early years of the 20th century. There was a leather, brass-studded, armchair on either side of the fireplace, with soft velvet, feather-filled, seat-cushions. In those days furniture was made to last a lifetime and it did in my parents' generation. It was certainly solid furniture that had been bought when my parents married, and much of it was in regular use for around sixty years until my father died in 1982.

A large gramophone cabinet stood in the alcove on one side of the chimneybreast. My parents had a number of records of popular classics as well as some light music of the period, and obviously enjoyed listening to music. Wagner's "Tannhäuser" and parts of Schubert's "Unfinished Symphony" were favorites with my father during my childhood, and he particularly enjoyed the excitement of hearing Tchaikovsky's "1812 Overture" with the resounding cannons towards the end of the piece. One record of two old-fashioned popular songs comes to my mind, as my father often sang "Shepherd of the Hills, I hear you calling", or "I'm in love with Sheila O'Shay, and Sheila O'Shay loves me". As I listened to his pleasant tenor voice joining with that of the soloist on the record, I wondered whether that was how my Christian name was chosen? Some of the other old melodic ballads that were so popular in my parents' young days were also in their collection of records. "I Hear You Calling Me" and "Trees" sung by Richard Tauber, "The Four Indian Love Lyrics" and Peter Dawson singing "Ole' Man River" and "Boots". I still get a lot of pleasure when I recall these old, pleasant melodies with their sentimental words. They are unforgettable. We had a very old record - even for those days - of Caruso singing an operatic aria and an even older, fainter, celluloid one of Dame Nellie Melba, which produced such a faint, cracked sound that I was distinctly unimpressed. All these records and many others were often played by my father during my childhood and provoke happy memories.

There was always the vigorous turning of the handle to wind up the gramophone before playing each side of the disc (although that word was not used!) before my father carefully placed the needle into the groove. I also recollect the, not infrequent, necessity for some additional winding-up towards the end of a record, in order to prevent the music slowing down and sliding off key as the piece reached its climax. The gramophone cabinet filled the alcove on one side of our pale green modern tiled fireplace. A large old clock – perhaps a wedding present in 1920? - sat on top of a floor-standing needlework cabinet on the other side. The front of this cabinet opened to reveal two shallow shelves and a full width drawer. This was supposed to hold the various requirements for sewing, but I can only remember the drawer containing photos and odd items, with other knick-knacks filling the little shelves. This became one of my 'playthings' when I was young, turning out the drawer, tidying the shelves, looking at the photos, or sorting the oddments. An old sepia photo in this drawer showed my parents standing by the side of their first Austin Seven car at the bottom of Porlock Hill in Somerset. I am sure that my father told me he drove his little car in reverse gear up this I: 3-gradient hill in the 1920s! Porlock Hill is still quite a taxing hill to drive up, with the very steep incline, coupled with exceedingly acute bends. It must have been quite an achievement in an early Austin Seven motorcar.

There was a large Put-U-Up in the dining room, with a hard, padded leather seat and solid, wooden arms. It was a bulky piece of furniture and a very uncomfortable two-seater settee. At some time a split had developed in the leather seat that my father managed to repair. I may have had some involvement in this damage by putting too much pressure on one place as I kneeled on it to look out of the window. The Put-U-Up was in regular use as a bed some years later, but I always thought it an ugly piece of furniture.

Our dining room is the room I remember most and was really the living room. In my mind's eye I can recall one or two incidents when my mother was still at home. I can picture her sitting in one of the leather-studded, velvet-cushioned armchairs in front of the fire, listening to the wireless that sat on top of the gramophone and warming her legs in front of the flames and crackling coals. I have several memories involving us eating a meal at the dining table. One Wednesday afternoon (early-closing day for my father), my mother placed a bowl of winkles on the table. My parents were picking the little fish out of their shells with a pin and eating them with enjoyment - and bread and butter. I squirmed at the thought of putting these slimy, crinkly lumps of food into my mouth and refused to taste what they evidently relished. My mother cooked tripe and onions for dinner sometimes and this dish I did enjoy. She sometimes bought live eels from a tank outside the fish shop in Kenton High Street and they were cooked and eaten with a parsley sauce for dinner. I remember these unusual dishes being eaten at the dining table more than the traditional ones that I am sure she also cooked. Winkles, tripe and eels probably featured in her meals as a child in Rotherhithe, but were also popular, nutritious and cheap meals in my childhood.

Glass doors divided our dining room from the 'drawing room', but these were normally kept closed and the room was not often used. I can't remember a fire being lit in this room until some years after I was married, when it became my husband's and my living room. I faintly remember that it had large, old-fashioned heavy furniture when my parents first moved into the house. They must have 'up-graded', as one day a new carpet was delivered and an abstract-patterned carpet square was laid on the floor. One did not have fitted carpets in those days. A large, old chesterfield (sofa) disappeared and soon after came the delivery of two new, very up-to-date Berkeley armchairs, with firm, broad arms and adjustable backs. I guess they were the latest style of the mid-to-late 1930s. The design of these chairs was far more appropriate to the style of the house, but perhaps the familiarity and soft comfort of the old leather chairs in the front reception room was more appealing to them. The drawing room was where the 'best' furniture and possessions were kept and it was the custom to use it only when entertaining visitors or on special occasions. These special occasions are not in the forefront of my memory; there were not many of them. I have no memories of time spent in this room with my parents, but my father subsequently used one of the Berkeley armchairs until he died.

The china cabinet in the drawing room displayed our 'best' china, some wineglasses and a bottle of sherry or port! A few books sat on the bottom shelf - a Pear's Encyclopedia, a large, battered Nuttall's dictionary, an old Austin Seven Handbook, an up-to-date Ford Eight Handbook and one or two other books of reference. Apart from a copy of 'She' by Rider Haggard, I can't recall that my parents owned any other books.

My mother often played the piano in our drawing room. She had a collection of well-known classics and quite a lot of other pieces of music. I can remember her playing Rachmaninov's Prelude in C Sharp Minor and being very frightened as she told me a story surrounding this piece of music. As she played she said the music was about a man who had been placed in his coffin before he was dead and the coffin lid was nailed down while he was still breathing. She described the account of his frantic knocking on the sides of the coffin, his desperate attempts to attract attention and to be released. The music grew softer and slower as the dying man's knocking gradually became less insistent and he grew weaker and weaker. Eventually, at the end of the piece, with no breath left and no strength to continue, the man died and then there was silence from the piano keys! I think I was nearly scared to death too, and never hear this piece of music without associating it with the tale I had been told. What a strange tale to tell to a small girl! She played brighter music too and I recall singing along to the tune "There is a Tavern in the Town" from her book of National Songs.

Next to the piano was my mother's treadle Singer sewing machine. I spent many otherwise unoccupied hours of my childhood 'turning out' the deep wooden drawers at either side of the machine, finding little treasures with which to amuse myself - fiddling with the machine accessories (which I am sure were rarely used), sorting the button box, tidying the cotton reels and messing about with various other oddments. A little oilcan was kept in one of the drawers and I can still almost smell the combination of wood, metal and sewing machine oil that met my nose when opening a drawer. The sewing machine itself could be slung down when not in use, leaving a smooth polished surface that was covered with a 'runner' made by my mother, using material of the same pattern as the Berkeley armchairs. (A similar 'runner' was placed diagonally across the dining table too, with an ashtray for my father at one end and a vase of flowers - or just a vase - in the middle.)

I have faint memories of my mother making curtains for the new house as she sat at her sewing machine, deftly moving the iron treadle to and fro with her feet. She also made shaped pelmets for all the main rooms, cutting them out of stiff card before covering them with the curtain material and finally stitching braid around the borders. I presume my father fitted the pelmets above the curtains, but I would not be surprised if my mother fixed these also. I have a feeling that she was a very versatile and practical lady when she was well. I believe she was good at needlework, but I am afraid I have not inherited her talent. She did not have much opportunity to pass on her skills to me.

As I look around the walls of my present home and see the variety of pictures and the many ornaments we now possess, our bookcases and shelves of books, I realize how easy it is today to buy paintings, all kinds of accessories and ornaments to decorate our homes. Bookshops tempt one in every shopping mall, but there were no pictures in any of the rooms in my childhood home and we had hardly any books. One or two mirrors hung on the walls, and a pair of the fashionable 1920s 'Oriental' vases was placed on either side of the mantelpiece in the two reception rooms. They were probably wedding presents. This was my childhood home, with a number of contrasts in modernity as opposed to traditional style, modern convenience and making-do. My parents were what one would term lower middle class, but were 'upwardly mobile' if my mother's illness had not overtaken their developing prosperity and happiness. Apart from the periods when I was again living with other people, it was my home from 1935 until I was in my early thirties.

We lived together in this house for only four years before my mother had her final nervous breakdown, so even if they were able, they did not have much opportunity to add any decorative features to their home. My father didn't buy any further embellishments for the home after my mother went into hospital in the summer of 1939; non-essential goods were unavailable during the War years and for some years afterwards, but I think he was reluctant to have luxuries – or even good holidays - that my mother was unable to share.

As I look back to when my husband and I moved into our first house in the early 1960s, I recall that our home was also devoid of any pictures for a number of years before we could afford to buy our first reproduction of an oil painting by Sisley. For years the local Library provided our family with most of the books we read. Books, decorative ornaments, paintings and reproductions of every style and period - price - were not readily available to the majority of ordinary folk until comparatively recent years. How times have changed!

Chapter Three

FAMILY BACKGROUND

Having described my parents' last home together, I feel I should add some colour and detail to their early years at the turn of the nineteenth and the beginning of the twentieth century. They were both born on the south bank of the River Thames, where ships sailed up to the Capital from all over the world to what was then the heart of London's dockland. My father was born in Bermondsey in 1894. He was an only child. His father was a lighterman on the Thames, rowing one of the flat-bottomed boats that carried cargo from the big ships anchored mid-stream in the deeper water of the River. The lighters were maneuvered alongside the ships, loaded up and then rowed to the wharves and warehouses, where their shipment was unloaded. It was extremely hard, strenuous work, requiring great strength and fitness, as well as skill in manhandling these heavily laden boats.

My father never understood why his own father had taken on this type of work, but I have tracked down that his grandfather was a lighterman in Bradford in Yorkshire and according to the 1881 census; his great-grandfather had also been a lighterman. The eldest son followed his father's occupation for at least three generations, but, thankfully, my own father broke with tradition and didn't follow in his father's footsteps. My grandfather's younger brothers had quite different careers: one became a Probation Officer, another an Accountant and the other two were both 'white collar' office workers and were quite comfortably off.

The hard manual work of rowing the cargo-laden boats required great strength and was too much for my grandfather, who tragically died at the age of thirty-seven. My father was only seven years old. He once told me that the only memory he had of his father was a recollection of the sensation of feeling his gnarled hands, hardened from heaving on the oars of his boat on the River Thames. He was told that his father had a heart attack or a fatal stroke while rowing, was brought to the quayside and pronounced dead. He had been made a 'Freeman of the River', but the River cost him his life.

Subsequent existence was hard for my grandmother. At the turn of the nineteenth century there was little or no assistance for widows, perhaps not even a pension, no child allowance, no social security, little opportunity of agreeable work, so no certainty of regular income. One of my father's 'white-collar-worker' uncles advised my grandmother to move from the flat she rented in Bermondsey, to Southend in Essex, where this Uncle Percy lived. He helped her to find a small house to rent, and she took in lodgers to earn enough money to provide for herself and for my father. As I was growing up my father occasionally spoke of his early life, telling me about how poor they were, of times when he didn't have any shoes to wear. If ever he was invited out to tea his mother gave him suet pudding to eat beforehand, to take the edge off his appetite. She did not want him to disgrace her by eating too much! That generation was very proud and self-
reliant - they had to be. My father was extremely thin all his life; maybe this was a legacy of the lean days of his childhood.

My grandmother took on an additional family responsibility when her late husband's niece, Lily, came to live with them after her mother died of tuberculosis. After the death of his wife, her husband had felt unable to cope and had left the family home. Auntie Lily, as I later knew her, and her two sisters May and Dolly, thus became orphans. Three relatives unofficially adopted the three sisters and my widowed grandmother took Lily into her poor home. I know that my father was very fond of his cousin and thought of her as a sister. After she married and had a daughter my parents often visited these relatives and when I was very young we had day-trips together to the seaside. This Aunt and Uncle had a great sense of humour and we seemed to be laughing and joking whenever we visited them. Auntie Lily was renowned for getting the giggles if she had a small glass of wine, and she was very amusing. I don't remember anything about the heated political conversations my mother reputedly had with my Uncle Jack, only the fun and the laughter. Sometimes I stayed with this Aunt and Uncle when my mother was unwell. I had a week's 'holiday' with them during school holidays during the War. I loved these periods with them in Coulsdon, playing in the little wooden summerhouse in their lovely garden that backed on to the Surrey hills, and can recall the beautiful sweet peas my Uncle used to grow. I felt somewhat in awe of my cousin Daphne, who seemed very grown-up to me.

My father had two cousins, who also lived in Southend-on-Sea during his childhood, but he lost touch with them over the years and I never knew them. He used to tell me of how he and these cousins, Bert and George, formed a little 'gang' when they were children. They played with their friends on the cliffs of Southend and Westcliff in the early days of the last century, before the area was developed into a popular seaside resort. The cliffs had not been landscaped and the seasonal illuminations of 'Never-Never-Land' had not yet become a visitor attraction. These young lads had a coded whistle, which they used to communicate with each other in their games. (Today, I suppose it would be a text message on a mobile!) Their whistle was passed down to my generation and became a very useful means of recognition between my father and I in later years. We were able to locate each other in crowds and elsewhere by whistling our little tune. Its short, distinctive rhythm and melody was immediately picked up and I knew the direction in which to go to find my father.

This whistle has now passed through three generations, as my husband and I used it with our own children when they were young. If we were on a family walk in the country or at the seaside, and our boys had wandered out of sight, the family signal carried well in the open air and helped us all to locate the whereabouts of each other. My husband and I still use the family whistle if we get separated in crowded shopping malls and find it very useful. It is a tiny bit of the past that is still valid. How amazed my father and his cousins would have been to know that their childhood gang whistle was still in regular use one hundred years later!

My father's education at a Board School ended as soon as he was legally able to leave school at thirteen and help his mother 'make ends meet'. He passed on to me one small memory of his schooldays, which he said almost made him wince as he related it. He could vividly recall the horrible sound of all his classmates scraping against their slates in the schoolroom with whatever they did their writing and figures with. He said that this harsh, rasping, grating, scraping sound was unforgettable. Life must have been hard for him and he seems to have remembered the 'hard' sensations - gnarled hands and grating on slates.

He did not have the opportunity of any further full-time education, although he went to what he called 'night school'- we would call it an evening class nowadays - as a young man. Although his formal education was very limited, he was a very cultured man, speaking well-constructed, always grammatical, sentences, in a pleasant-toned voice. From time to time in my childhood he would burst forth into reciting poetry or excerpts from Shakespeare in quite dramatic tones.... "Friends, Romans, countrymen, lend me your ears, I come to bury Caesar, not to praise him..." or "Spanish ships of war at sea, I have sighted fifty-three!", and other similar passages. He knew a lot of poetry and while doing a job around the house I would catch the sound of him reciting with some fervour... "Oh to be in England, now that April's here", or lines from the 'Charge of the Light Brigade' – "guns to the left of them, guns to the right of them, volleyed and thundered". I have no idea where he had heard all this poetry or studied Shakespeare, but assume he had attended Literature Classes at his Night School. I often overheard him singing snatches of songs when I was young - parts of operatic arias, or some of the old ballads of which he seemed to know so many. I can still hear him in my mind singing, "Softly awakes my heart..." from Samson and Delilah, or "I'll sing thee songs of Araby" or one or another of the popular songs of the period such as "We fly through the air with the greatest of ease, a man and a girl on a flying trapeze". His repertoire was wide!

He was called up during the First World War and joined the Royal Naval Air Service. His War service was spent on barrage balloon stations in the Orkney Islands, where Scapa Flow was a Naval Base. He did not pass his medical examination with A1 grade and perhaps he was posted to these Scottish Islands because he was not fit enough for front-line service. Although of average height, he was extremely thin, was not a robust man, and never weighed more than eight-and-a-half stone in his life. I think he saw active service in defence of the Grand Fleet as it sailed from Scapa Flow to the Battle of Jutland in 1916, but his life was not seriously endangered on the battlefield. He observed the scuttling of the German Fleet in Scapa Flow just after the end of the War and I found two old, faded picture postcards among his memorabilia that show the ships as they sank into the sea.

He exchanged Christmas cards for many years with one or two old comrades, but they didn't write letters to each other and they never met again; I learned little about his years in the Forces. He kept what he called his 'ditty box' for the rest of his life, and told me that this small wooden box contained all his personal documents during his service years, but I only remember it as a container for brushes and tins of polish for cleaning his shoes. He had used the same brushes to clean his boots when he was in the Forces! I learned nothing about his wartime experiences.

There were not many career opportunities early in the twentieth century for the majority of youngsters who received merely a basic education. There was little industry in Southend, but on leaving school my father told me he was lucky enough to get his first job in a men's clothing shop in the town. Some time later he obtained a better position in London, left home, found lodgings in South London, and began working in a branch of 'Meakers', a high-class men's outfitters' shop. This firm had many branches in the South of

England. He worked in two of their biggest London shops, first in Holborn and later had promotion to the position of 'first man' (Assistant Manager?) in their large shop in Piccadilly. Soon after he came out of the Forces at the end of the First World War he became Manager of Meakers' new branch that opened in Ealing Broadway. He remained in this position until his retirement. He once told me that he thought he would have had further promotion within the company had it not been for my mother's mental illness, with all the associated worry and anxiety that prevented him from taking on extra responsibility. Further promotion did not come his way.

My father's Uncle Percy (after whom he was named and who had advised his mother to move to Southend) married my mother's much older sister Alice Scott, and this introduced the two families of Scott and Brook to each other. My parents marriage brought about an unusual dual relationship, as these relatives became their brother and sister-in-law, (Alice and 'Perce') as well as their Aunt Alice and Uncle Percy. My father was twenty-six years old and my mother was two years younger when they married in 1920 and their first home was in the flat over the new Meakers Menswear shop in Ealing Broadway. Although I never went into the flat, I saw the external iron staircase behind the shop that led up to their first home when I was a small child. Some years later they moved to their first house at Osterley.

I recollect many details of the shop itself, with its long, curved, plate-glass windows arcading through to the shop door. I can recall my father spending many hours throughout his working life in meticulously dressing the windows of this long double frontage. Meakers shops were well known for their elaborate and detailed window displays, showing examples of most of their merchandise. Window-dressing periods - especially for the Christmas display when a sample of every kind of clothing or object suitable for giving as a Christmas gift had to be on show - were very time-consuming and anxious periods for my father. Cuff-links or tie pins in attractive boxes, ties and socks in abundance, Bonsoir pyjamas, hats of every style, variously patterned wool scarves, soft leather Dent's gloves, boxes of fine cotton Pyramid handkerchiefs and Van Heusen shirts were all displayed amongst 'sports' jackets and more expensive clothing, to tempt the window-shopper to step inside.

It was a very long shop, with elegantly styled, oak-framed, plate glass counters displaying trays of shirts, ties, handkerchiefs and gloves beneath. Deep oak drawers ranged behind the counters held discreetly concealed underwear. There was an old-fashioned cash register, with a bell that rang harshly when the till was opened. Half way up on the right side of the shop was a brick fireplace with large mirrors fitted behind it and mirror-fronted cupboards at either side. An open coal fire burned all day during the cold winter months. It looked wonderfully cheering to the customers and provided pleasant warmth for anyone standing in front of it, but must have produced a lot of dust and dirt. The shop assistants were not allowed to stand in front of the fire, but always had to be busy - or look busy - tidying stock, dusting shelves, or waiting expectantly behind the counters, even if they were not serving customers. They also had to clean out the ashes from the grate each morning, then prepare and light a fresh fire. There was no heating in the work place until this coal fire began to blaze.

There was a rotating display fixture for 'sports' jackets near the rear of the shop. I used to like swinging this bit of equipment around when I was a small child if I was occasionally in the shop with my mother waiting for closing time, when we could all go home together in the car. (I believe this same carousel is now displaying items of clothing in another men's outfitters in Ealing!)

A large area at the far end of my father's shop extended to the right and was used exclusively for bespoke (made-to-measure) suits. An oak-framed, free-standing, glass display cabinet was in the middle of this space, upon which my father carefully set down heavy bolts of cloth before unrolling them for customers to handle and select their material for a new tailored suit. I can picture my father measuring a customer for a suit, with his tape-measure hanging around his neck, then dexterously moving it along his customer's arms, chest, waist, inside and outside leg, carefully noting each measurement for the tailor. The gleaming, reflecting doors of a number of mirror-walled fitting rooms were all around the sides of this spacious area and one of these - the tiny corner one - was used by the staff for their tea breaks. It was always called the 'cubby-hole' because it was so small, with sufficient space for only one adult to have their coffee or tea break. An electric fire was laid on its back in order to stand the kettle on top to boil the water.

Another part of the shop I remember well and squirm as I think of it was called 'out the back', where the polished parquet flooring suddenly changed to rough stone as one opened another mirrored doorway leading to the toilet and washing facilities - if such they could be called. A large, rather dirty, crazed butler sink was situated in a corner, with only one tap from which the kettle was filled with cold water for tea, and later the tap was turned on again to rinse the used cups. I doubt that they were ever washed properly! A rough wooden door opposite the old sink opened on to a rather squalid toilet. This small utility area was lit by one bare electric light bulb. Neither of these very basic facilities, nor the dangerous use of the electric fire, would pass health and safety regulations today.

'Out the back' was such a contrast to the large expanse of fine, light-oak, flooring in the shop, the smart light fittings and the immaculate appearance of the entire shop, which was cleaned by the Staff - who looked equally immaculate in their navy blue, three-piece suits. The floor was regularly polished, the glass counters and oak shelves were dusted every day, and all the mirrored doors were always gleaming. Mirrors and glass featured everywhere and everything was bright and shining. (The young male shop assistants were very well trained in these domestic duties and should have been more than competent to help their wives in future days.)

In a retirement letter to my father in 1961, the company's founder, Mr. Ben Meaker, recalled my father's fifty years of service to Meakers. He wrote, "My dear Brook, Your retirement to me is like parting with an old friend. We have experienced some very stirring times over the many years, two world Wars. I think it was when I returned from America in 1919 that the Ealing shop was the first one that I fitted out with American ideas which I gleaned whilst over there. It was the beginning of our up to date shop fitting. We were copied in all directions by all and sundry. I have nothing but happy memories of you as one of our stalwart youngsters." (Sic)

My father was manager of the Ealing Broadway branch for about forty years, but had worked for the firm for about fifty years. After these many years of service mentioned in the letter from Mr. Meaker, his official pension was minimal, but in recognition of his long period of loyal service it was increased to the princely sum of £520 a year. He was also given a television set - his first - as a retirement present. A lifetime's work with one company, with such loyal service is unusual nowadays. His pride in the receipt of this personal letter in recognition of his long service, together with the hours of pleasure my father had in watching his television in his retirement were enhanced by the delight he had in having such a gift. He was grateful for his (slightly) enhanced pension. Golden handshakes were unknown in that era. A little appreciation went a long way and contentment seemed easier to find in the midst of difficulty in a less acquisitive and demanding society.

Company pension schemes were not common in the years before the Second World War and Meakers only started their pension scheme after the War had ended, so my father had only contributed for a few years before he reached retirement age. He continued working until he was sixty-seven in order to increase his pension a little. He lived comfortably, but modestly, for a further twenty years, by which time Meakers as a Company had disappeared from the High Streets. Nobody in the family wished to carry on the business after Mr. Ben Meaker died, so sadly 'Meakers' Men's Outfitters' no longer exists. Its distinctive logo of a spreading oak tree, signifying reliability, good quality merchandise and excellent service has faded from the public's memory.

My father very rarely had a day off work for sickness or any other reason, and went into work to open up the shop and let the staff in on time even when he was sometimes very unwell, the weather was appalling and public transport almost at a standstill. I can recall only two occasions when he was unable to get to work at all. He had 'flu at some time during the War and it seemed so strange to find him at home, in bed, downstairs on our put-u-up, when I came home from school. The other occasion was after the War had ended. He had an accident on the road as he traveled to Ealing on his motorised bicycle - a Minimotor - and was in hospital with concussion for some time.

During heavy snow in winter, the Air Raids in the Blitz, and the V1s, V2s towards the end of the War, he made sure that he was at work by 9 a.m. in order to unlock the shop. He never took time off to visit my mother in Hospital, but only visited her on a Sunday afternoon. I don't know how he coped in earlier years when she began to have early symptoms of her mental illness.

Long ago my father told me that his mother had died in 1924 while living with my parents. After his death I discovered that this was the same year in which Peggy died, so my father lost his mother and his first daughter in the same year. I found her funeral Memorial card when rummaging around in the drawer of the needlework cabinet as a child. I didn't understand who it referred to then, but I read it again years later: 'Good was her heart, in friendship sound; Patient in pain and loved by all around; Her pain is o'er, her grief for ever done, A life of everlasting joy she's now begun.' I almost felt that I knew her a little from these words. She had been widowed for twenty-three years and had had a very hard life.

My mother was born in Rotherhithe, close to the Surrey Commercial Docks. Her parents lost three children in infancy and she was the youngest of five surviving children. Her father was known as a wood merchant, and he supplied firewood to a large area of South London. He bought the cheap, rough wood from the cargoes of timber that came up the River from Sweden to the Surrey Docks. The better quality wood was bought by furniture manufacturers or for use in the building industry. There was a great demand for firewood in the late nineteenth and early twentieth centuries, and my grandfather seized the opportunity of developing his own business in this basic commodity. The 1881 census informs me that he employed five men, nine women and five boys in his business. The women chopped the wood into small sticks and the boys tied these into bundles in a building he had erected at the bottom of the 'yard' behind their home in Paradise Street, a short road that ran parallel to Jamaica Road and the River. I presume the men did the heavy sawing of the timber and perhaps helped to deliver the firewood. In her old age my mother told me that my grandfather had stabling for horses in their yard at the back of the house, that he owned several carts and horses, and also some handcarts. He traded with most of the oil shops and iron merchants in South London supplying them with their stocks of firewood. When I visited my mother in hospital when she was quite elderly, she sometimes referred to her past, reminiscing over being occasionally taken around the streets in a horse and cart with her father when she was a girl. She also told me that they kept a cow at some time in their back yard, together with chickens and some rabbits.

Her father became quite a wealthy man and I understand that he was the landlord of most of the houses in Paradise Street. He was reputed to have a very short temper and was also a heavy drinker. The two facts are no doubt linked! Either he or my great-grandfather rowed on the Thames in the Doggetts Coat and Badge Race. This is an ancient and once very famous rowing competition, which claimed to be the longest-running sporting event in the world! I imagine it now has the least publicity and the smallest interest - if indeed the Race still occurs. An actor named Thomas Doggett began the race for newly qualified Watermen in the early part of the eighteenth century. It was first rowed in 1715; together with prize money, the winner was given a coat and a badge emblazoned with the White Horse of Hanover. It was a race for tough men, who rowed against the tide in wherries, which were stronger, heavier craft than present-day rowing boats. If my grandfather did row in it, it must have been in his youth; he looks an un-athletic man in the family group photograph taken at my parents' wedding. Although my father's father was a Freeman of the River, I never heard that he rowed in this ancient race.

Unlike my father, my mother grew up in a comfortably off family. My only first cousin, who was a bridesmaid at my mother's wedding, but who is not even of my generation, and whom I have rarely met, gave me a written description of my mother's childhood home, remembered from her father's youth. The living rooms were quite lavishly furnished in an early Victorian style and the family sitting room was on the first floor. Her father told her that as well as the ornate and somewhat opulent furniture and furnishings, there was a grand piano that was only used on special occasions. But my mother and her sister, Ada must surely have learned to play on this instrument, as both had a piano in their homes, both had quite large collections of music and I know my mother played reasonably well. Brother Albert (my almost-unknown cousin's father) was a bus driver in Catford, with a passion for greyhound racing, and he was possibly more interested in this than noticing his little sister playing the piano. He was many years older than my mother and had probably left home and was married by the time she was old enough to sit on a piano stool. There was so much music stacked in our piano stool when I was young that I feel sure that my mother must have been taught to play on the grand piano in her childhood.

A large ground floor room in the house had been converted into a meeting room and let out to a Mission. No doubt my grandfather had found another source of income to add to the rents he collected and the firewood he delivered! He must have been quite an entrepreneur in the late nineteenth and early twentieth centuries. My mother told me when she was very old that she used to go to a Mission meeting, called 'The Ark' when she was a girl. She didn't say that this meeting was held in her own home, so I shall never know whether the ground floor mission room and 'The Ark' were one and the same. Apparently this meeting room was used for my parents' wedding reception and no doubt that of her two sisters also, but my father never spoke of it.

My grandmother did all the cooking for her family on an open range in a very tiny kitchen in this seemingly quite large house. There was no indoor water supply and she had to go into the 'yard' for all the water required for cooking, washing and all the family needs. The domestic facilities seem to have been quite primitive and I believe my grandmother had a hard life. She died after contracting an infection in a cut on her hand when opening a tin of food. Septicemia developed within a few days and she died quite suddenly.

I know nothing at all about my mother's eldest brother and I have no memory of ever meeting my greyhound-race-loving Uncle Albert. These two uncles and their two sisters, Alice and Ada, were many years older than my mother, Lily, who was very much of an afterthought! My grandmother was forty-five years old when my mother arrived on the scene in 1896, an 'elderly' mother indeed in those times, and one much worn down with child-bearing and the harshness of her life. My mother was expected to help her ageing mother with the household chores after she left school and didn't go out to work until the First World War began.

Women had to take their share in the War effort when the men had gone to the Front and my mother was then able to, hopefully, have a little independence, a job, friendship, and perhaps some money of her own. Until then it had been presumed that as she was the youngest daughter, she would stay at home and help with the running of the household. Her sisters had grown up, married and left home, but in those days (and even in my youth) girls didn't leave home until marriage; they were more or less literally "given away" at their marriage service. In view of her subsequent, apparently strong, political views, I feel she could have become involved in the Suffragette Movement if she had had the opportunity!

Maybe my Aunts were keen to move away from the Surrey Docks, the firewood and perhaps their tough father! Ada married a schoolteacher and moved to Bromley, then to Beckenham. Alice married my father's Uncle Percy who worked in the City and travelled into London each day from Southend. Neither my Auntie Ada nor my Auntie Alice had any children. Uncle 'Perce' and my Auntie Alice did not figure much in my life, although I stayed with them once when I was a small child, perhaps to give my mother a break. I can remember sitting at their breakfast table, in their rather 'posh' dining room and having half a grapefruit put in front of me, together with a small, pointed silver spoon. We had always eaten Libby's tinned grapefruit at home; I didn't know how to tackle this fruit with the flesh still attached to the thick skin and I struggled away, trying not to be noticed as I picked at it with my fingers.

Both my mother's sisters were very 'correct' in their speech and behaviour, very genteel, and neither they, nor my mother had any sign of their London origins and it would seem that they were very carefully brought up. To my childish mind they dressed very fashionably in the nineteen-thirties and were very 'ladylike'! I knew of no cousins apart from Daphne and did not know of the existence of my first cousin, Joyce, until I attended her father's (my unknown Uncle Albert's) funeral when I was about forty. She is my informant concerning our mutual grandparents.

My mother's mother died, aged sixty-nine, only two months after my parents were married. Her funeral Memorial Card was also among various papers in the old needlework cabinet, and on the front it says, "At Rest". This phrase seemed very appropriate for her, as I believe she had little rest during her lifetime. My grandfather died three years later. I am told that he was overcome with grief at his wife's sudden death and apparently drank away the sorrows of his bereavement along with the profits of his business interests.

Perhaps he had nobody to restrain his excesses after his wife had died. He lost interest in his successful business and his property concerns, and soon all his money had gone. His surviving children, Albert, Alice, Ada and my mother were left nothing – except perhaps some debts!

My parents were still living in the flat over the shop when their first baby was born. They had a very distressing period during Peggy's short life. My father never spoke to me about the loss of three parents, together with the death of his first daughter in such a comparatively short space of time. Those four years were filled with sorrow and loss. My maternal grandmother's death, so shortly after my parents' marriage was followed by the birth of their handicapped daughter, who died in 1924, the same year in which my paternal grandmother died. My mother's father had died the previous year. What a sad time my parents had in the first few years of their marriage.

When visiting my elderly mother in hospital some time after my father had died, I once asked her if she remembered how she felt when she knew the seriousness of Peggy's condition. She replied, "Well, I thought, that's your lot my girl; you've just got to put up with it!" but she had nobody with experience of children to turn to for support. She had been used to a hard life at home and Peggy was born so soon after her own mother had died. My mother then talked to me a little of this sister I never knew. She told me that Peggy had suffered many fits nearly every day. One day, so my mother said, Peggy was so bad that she carried her in her arms to the doctor, who immediately admitted the baby to hospital, where she died three days later. My mother said to me, "I cannot understand why, after I had looked after her for so long, they took Peggy away on a Friday and by the Monday she was dead. I cannot understand it." As she said this, she rocked her arms and shook her head in incomprehension over what had occurred over sixty years previously.

I don't know how true these details are, as my mother was old and mentally ill, but she was able to talk quite rationally and sensibly about many things, particularly those relating to her early years. I have found no bereavement card in memory of Peggy, no photos of her, or mementos of any kind among my father's papers. If I had not asked about the meaning of the word "Peggy" that I had seen engraved on the tea caddy spoon many years ago, I think I would never have known of her sad, short existence.

I knew nothing about my grandparents or of their lives or deaths while my parents were alive, and have only discovered the close proximity of these relatives' deaths whilst researching for this book. Was this early history recorded on my mother's medical notes, or known by the various Doctors who attended her? Did anyone ever talk to her about these distressing experiences?

I doubt whether either of my parents were able to express their grief and unhappiness at the loss of their first daughter. There was certainly no bereavement counseling in those long ago days and the usual advice was "least said, soonest mended" so I doubt whether it was talked over with friends and relations. Their sorrow was kept very much to themselves. My parents were probably expected to 'forget' their daughter Peggy, just as I was expected to 'forget' my mother. My father never talked to me about Peggy or about my mother after she went into Hospital; maybe his sorrow was unspeakable. It would seem that my mother internalised her grief at her mother's sudden death, followed to soon by her daughter's, and this may have subsequently expressed itself in her own mental illness. To experience the deaths of three parents and one baby daughter in the space of four years must have brought immense sorrow and distress into both of their lives. I remember my father as a very reserved person and I believe that my mother was not very self-confident; perhaps they were unable to comfort each other. I am sure that my Auntie Ada and Uncle Bert were my parents' greatest support, even if it was unspoken. My mother always referred to him very warmly as her "brother Bert" in her old age, although he was in fact her brother-in-law, but she could - or would - not believe that he was therefore my Uncle. I remember him, too, as a very kind and gentle, yet formal and restrained, man.

My parents may have thought it unwise to risk a second pregnancy with the fear of another disabled child, or a recurrence of my mother's depression. They may also have been concerned about starting a family again during the worrying years of the Depression. They may have just enjoyed the good social times of the 'roaring twenties' with their sisters- and brothers-in-law. They were three childless couples and I am sure that my arrival was a shock. When visiting my mother in Hospital I once asked about this and she told me, "I didn't know I'd fallen, my girl!"

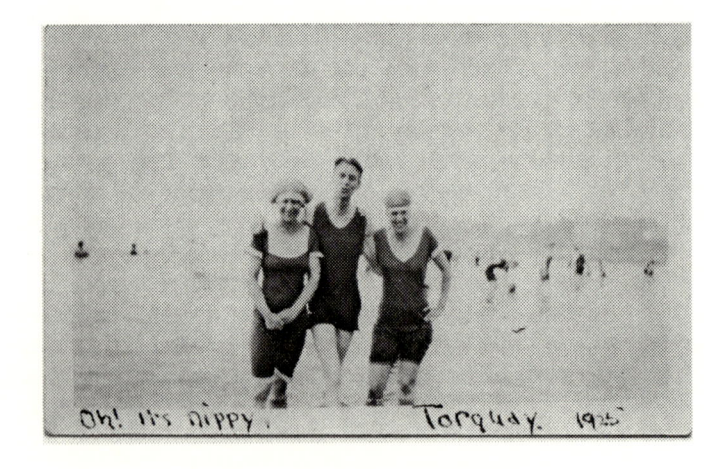

Three 'bathing beauties'

They also had good times with my father's cousin Lily and her husband. They had touring holidays in the Lake District in their little car, days at the seaside and even had a holiday abroad, cruising along the River Rhine with my elderly 'Uncle' and 'Auntie' Connell, whose actual relationship to me was always unclear. I have photos of my parents on these holidays with their various relations and they seemed happy and well. My father told me that they used to go to concerts at the Queen's Hall in Langham Place, which was destroyed in the London Blitz in 1941. These Concerts were inaugurated and conducted by Sir Henry Wood at the turn of the century and were first performed in the Queen's Hall. They were the forerunners of the annual Promenade Concerts at the Royal Albert Hall in London. It would appear that life was good to them for a few years.

They were especially close to my Auntie Ada and Uncle Bert and there were many visits between the two sisters and their husbands. It was fashionable to play Whist in those pre-TV days and I know that my parents played cards with these relatives - can I remember them sitting around the card table when I was small? I think I can. My father did not read or play music, but he had a lovely voice, as did my Uncle Bert, who had been a choirboy in his youth, and I am sure there were 'sing-songs' and home entertainment round the piano during these years. I can imagine solos or duets being sung with my mother or aunt at the piano and one or another of the men, or my parents, singing together. Many of these songs are still familiar to me – "Just a Song at Twilight", "You Are My Heart's Delight" "Because God Made You Mine" - as I can recall my father singing them at home. They must have brought bittersweet memories to him when he sang them on his own in later years. All these songs originated long before my generation, but I sometimes find myself singing a few lines, just as he spontaneously sang them during my childhood.

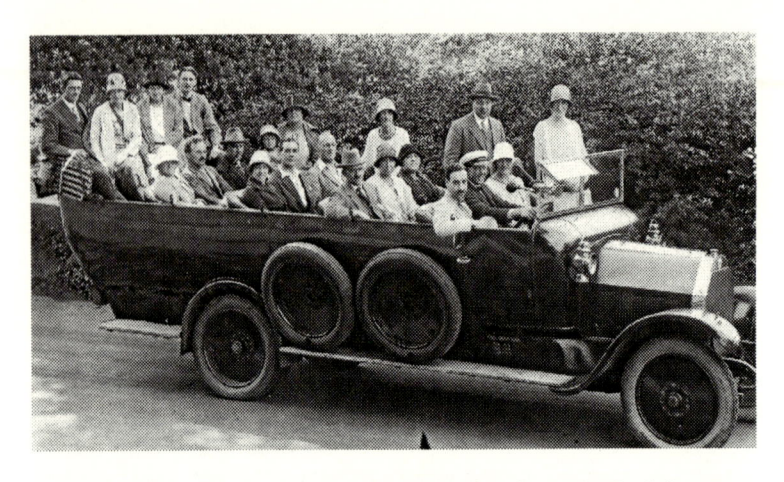

My parents, aunt and uncle on the back seat of a 'char-a-banc'

The circumstances of my parents' early lives were very different from those of my own childhood, but there are similarities. My father's early bereavement and moving away from the area of his birth resemble my own loss of my mother, not by death, but by illness and our move to a new neighborhood. I had quite a lot of responsibility in the home as I grew up, somewhat mirroring my mother's experience. All my recollections of my father at home during my childhood and in later years, are of a reserved man with an uncomplaining nature and an even temper, with a brightness and gaiety that seemed overlaid with tenseness and anxiety. He was always neat and smart in his appearance, very independent, but without supportive friends or relations as he grew older. After my mother's last major illness in 1939 he seemed a very lonely man for the rest of his life, but he responded stoically and cheerfully to all the sadness he had experienced. I think I had a measure of loneliness in my life too; perhaps – I hope - I too have inherited his cheerful nature.

I remember only one occasion during my childhood when my father (understandably) showed anger. It was not very long after he had employed a housekeeper to care for us. For a little while I had no bedroom of my own and had to sleep on a makeshift bed on the floor of my father's room. Our housekeeper's daughter and I had locked his bedroom door one Saturday evening in a childish bit of mischief, to prevent me from going to bed at the usual time. Our plan was to have a 'midnight feast' in her bedroom - before her mother came to bed! When my father came home from work late on the Saturday evening, I was told it was time for bed and we two girls couldn't find the key, trying to delay my bedtime. Eventually, we realised that we had truly lost the key and late in the evening he had to set to and force the lock to open his bedroom door. He was tired after a long day's work, but neither he nor I could go to bed until the door was opened. He grew very frustrated and consequently angry, and it is the only time in my life that I remember him losing patience and hearing him swear – and then it was only a mild 'Damn!' as he tried to force the lock. I was shocked! Rose and I didn't have our 'feast'. I have no idea what delicacies or treats we presumed we would be able to find in a larder whose shelves were not exactly brimming over with goodies, or even spare basic foods, in 1940.

My father had one or two sayings that he quoted to me when they seemed to him to be applicable, especially about cleaning my bike as I grew up! I clearly remember hearing, "If a job's worth doing, it's worth doing well" "Procrastination is the thief of time," and I am sure they have influenced the way I go about my day-to-day life.

Chapter Four

HAPPY DAYS!

Between the periods of sadness in their lives, my parents had many enjoyable outings and holidays in my father's Austin Seven car in the years both before and after my birth. There were some jolly times with the aunts and uncles, my cousin Daphne and family friends before we moved from Osterley. I have a number of old photos that were taken at the seaside during some of these day trips and I can look at a group of relatives sitting on the beach eating ice cream cornets. My cousin Daphne is in the picture and I appear to be little more than a toddler, seated on the sand with a large beach ball between my knees. Two photos show everyone wearing unglamorous and hideous-looking swimsuits; my father and two uncles pose in their one-piece, torso-covering, black bathing costumes, with straps over the shoulders - no men's trunks or briefs in those days - and my cousin and I are paddling and making sandcastles. I am clad in a hideous hand-knitted costume with a broad stripe in contrasting wool across my chest. Everyone looks so happy and relaxed in these old pictures, but I find that reviewing them revives no memories of the occasions, the people, the atmosphere, or the fun that we all apparently had.

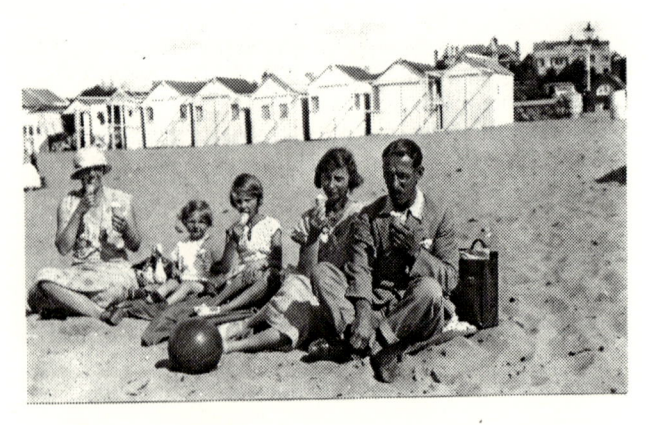

With my mother, my cousin and her parents.

My father was driving the little old Austin Seven home one summer Sunday evening after a long day spent on the beach. My mother sat in the passenger seat at his side and I was curled up in the back, supposedly dozing off to sleep. The happenings of the day are completely forgotten, but I very clearly recall my hand sliding up to fiddle with a sharp split in the celluloid window. My fingers could not resist the temptation to creep up and pick at the crack, and, I fear, to make it worse. The window was yellowed, the celluloid was brittle and not very clear, and the back seat was hard. The poor suspension in cars in those days made sleeping while travelling rather difficult. It was more interesting to tamper with the split in the window and make it larger. I could not have been more than four years old, but the memory is so vivid I can still almost feel the sharp, broken edges of the celluloid under my fingernail.

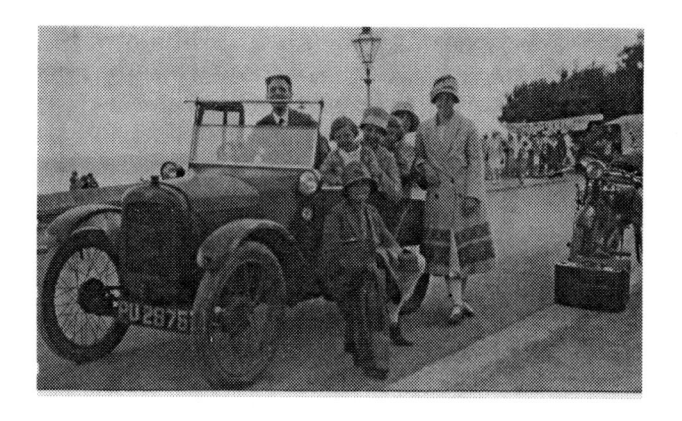

On the seafront in the Austin Seven

Days at the seaside may not have been as frequent after our move in 1935 to what were then the outer suburbs of north London. Our relatives lived in Kent and Surrey, and a drive to the coast was considerably further for us than for my aunts and uncles as we now had to get across London. Traffic congestion was not a problem in those days, but the tediousness of driving through London and the time that added to our journey, as the family car chugged at a leisurely pace along the roads, made a visit to the South coast a less frequent Sunday outing. Speed was not 'of the essence' in those days with pre-war motor vehicles and uncrowded roads.

A certain chocolate bar called 'Motoring Chocolate' was popular with my parents when I was young and no doubt with many others who had a car in those years. It was a plain chocolate bar containing large pieces of almonds and succulent whole raisins. I can imagine my parents driving along the quiet country lanes eating the silver-paper-wrapped chocolate. (I can remember having some too!) No car radio or heater in the car, no power steering or automatic gear change, no air conditioning or air bags, no automatic window adjustment or central locking, no crowded motorways or traffic-hold-ups, and no 'road rage'. There was just the excitement and dubious delight of cranking the starter handle, but being independent on the road, in control and free. Happy days indeed! Servicing the car and tinkering under the bonnet on Sunday mornings was my father's and many men's hobby. The question "How's the car going, Percy?" - and or Bert, or Jack, - was almost the first greeting when the relatives met.

The little Austin car came to the end of its serviceable life at about the same time that we moved to Kenton, and my father replaced it with a second-hand Ford 8 car - BMD 336. He drove it to work every day until shortly after the start of the War, when petrol rationing came into force. Our 'new' car then had to remain in the garage until my father eventually sold it at a loss. Who wanted to buy a car in wartime? Before selling the old 1926 Austin Seven he had removed the clock from the dashboard, and this crude little timepiece sat on the window-ledge in our kitchen for many, many years, keeping excellent time. It was supported on either side by two of my childhood toy bricks that had been stuck on to the window ledge, where it sat securely wedged between them. I think this little old clock was a memento for my father of happy touring holidays and excursions my parents had together before I was born, as well as our various outings and holidays during the early nineteen thirties. It was also a souvenir for my father of a much-loved little car from the early days of motoring.

He was an experienced driver before compulsory Driving Tests were introduced, never took a driving test and I know he enjoyed driving. He never had an accident and had only one traffic offence in the whole of his driving career. This was for omitting to notice a rather obscure red traffic light, sited almost under a railway bridge in South London. My father always commented on it when we drove under this particular bridge on our way to visit our relatives in Beckenham, carefully observing that the lights were green before proceeding. He was very dismayed that he had inadvertently spoiled his perfect record. He drove from early in the 1920s' right up until a few weeks before his death in 1982 (apart from a long period during the War and afterwards). He was unable to own a car again until 1956, when my husband and I shared the ownership of our first car - a second-hand pre-war Austin Cambridge – with my father!

In the years leading up to the War our periodic outings in the more modern Ford car continued occasionally on Wednesday afternoons (early closing day at the shop and a half-day holiday for my father) but more often on Sundays, until my mother's next 'nervous breakdown'. We visited Burnham Beeches, Maidenhead, Hurley Lock and other places along the Thames. We picnicked at the water's edge at Hurley and I remember paddling in the shallow water by the riverside. We drove to various beauty spots in Surrey - Frensham Ponds, Box Hill and the Devil's Punch Bowl - now rather overgrown and surrounded by busy roads and heavy traffic.

My parents had made friends with some of our new neighbours in Kenton who had a son about my age, named Keith. Our two families sometimes went out together on Wednesday afternoons in the school holidays. Keith's father was the Manager of a stationer's shop, so the two fathers had something in common and shared a Wednesday early-closing day each week. Mr. Reynolds' shop was in Pinner, near Harrow and on one occasion we all went to the annual Pinner Mop Fair, watched the procession wend its colourful, noisy way down the High Street. I remember the event clearly as we mingled with the crowds, enjoying the sideshows, the swing-boats and the entertainments.

Sadly for us all, this friendship between our families was cut short when Mr. Reynolds moved to another branch of his firm. This also meant that they moved from their attractive modern house next-door-but-one to ours, and I lost my friend Keith. They came back to visit at the time of King George VI's Coronation. Whilst his parents went up to London to join the crowds watching the Royal procession from the roadside, Keith was left to spend the night with us. He was going to sleep in my big back bedroom and share my bed. My mother placed a bolster in the middle of the bed, to keep it all 'respectable' and Keith and I spent the night together! We were very excited and chattered continually, so it was very late before we dropped off to sleep and even then we only slept for a little while.

Keith woke me early in the morning to tell me that his parents had brought chocolate medallions of the King and Queen for both of us. They had told my parents that these were to be given to us at the time of the Coronation, but no sooner. We made our way into my parents' bedroom in the small hours and pestered my mother and father, begging to be given our chocolate souvenirs before the Coronation Ceremony. I am sure we made rather a nuisance of ourselves and were more persuasive because there were two of us, and perhaps we succeeded in eating our chocolate long before breakfast. That's my only memory of the Coronation in 1937 and it is also the only time during my childhood or teenage years I had a friend staying overnight in my home. One didn't have 'sleep-overs' in those pre-war days, and Keith and I didn't meet again.

My parents had other friends living in Kenton. The husband was Manager of Burton's the Tailor's in Ealing Broadway, almost opposite Meakers. Mr. Brownbill had noticed the group of new houses being built in Kenton Lane as he drove to work each day in his little Morris car, and was responsible for suggesting the Harrow area to my father. Mr. and Mrs. Brownbill and our two families visited each other from time to time, but I cannot recall the adults using each other's first names. People were much more formal in their relationships then. They had two sons and also had an Airedale dog, and one year we also acquired a pedigree Airedale puppy. Mr. and Mrs. Brownbill had spent Christmas with relatives in their hometown of Liverpool, and they brought back a puppy from another litter for us. She was such a tiny puppy that Mrs. Brownbill managed to carry her in a 'holdall' on the train journey back to London. My parents named her Betty. She could hardly stagger around our dining room when we first had her, and was so small she could creep beneath the stretcher bars that extended between the legs of our dining table.

She soon grew into a big, strong dog, becoming quite difficult for my mother to control when we went out shopping. I think Betty had been bought as company for my mother while I was at school, possibly as therapy for her nerves. When my mother had to return to hospital a year or two later, poor Betty was left in the garden all day while my father was at work. There was nobody to look after her, train her, or take her for walks. She ran riot in the garden throughout the day, ruined the plants, roughed up the lawn and became yet another problem for my father to deal with.

Although we had fewer day trips to the coast after moving to Kenton, I well recall one holiday at the seaside. My parents were sitting on the beach with their backs against the promenade wall. The weather was cold and blustery and they didn't want to go bathing in the rather unwelcoming sea. I was clad in my (larger – or just stretched?) hand-knitted costume that still figured a broad diagonal contrasting stripe across my chest. How was this woolen garment expected to react when saturated with water? I can still remember the cold, clammy feeling as it clung to my nether regions after I had been in the sea. The cold, clinging dampness was horrible. I must have been a very keen bather as a little girl, to put on this awful bathing costume and go into the water on a cold day. I was eager to learn how to swim, but could not persuade my parents to join me in the water on this chilly afternoon. I remember a previous 'dip' in the sea, when my mother was supporting my efforts to swim by holding the back of my costume (the same ghastly striped one) as I dangled in the water, flapping my arms and legs. The vague memory brings back the sensation of the water-laden costume and my cold, damp behind! I had almost - but not quite - managed to stay afloat on that occasion and I was keen to get my 'sea legs' before the summer ended.

On this particular dull, breezy day however, neither my father nor my mother would even put their feet into the water. I still have quite a clear memory of the scene. I was playing about in the shallow water in my bathing costume, but longing to be able to go right into the sea and - to swim. My father told me to walk out into the deeper water, turn round and face him, then swim in with the waves. I took him at his word, did exactly as he said and waded out until I was in a good depth of water - for a five or six year old - then turned round and following my parent's encouraging words, I struck out. Doing my 'doggy paddle' or sort-of breaststroke I swam towards the shore as they sat watching me, huddled up in coats, counting each stroke, encouraging and urging me on. I successfully managed twenty-seven strokes and was extremely proud of my achievement.

I became a very enthusiastic and steady swimmer in the coming years, enjoying swimming in our local open-air unheated swimming pool with a good school friend and in the sea with my father on the holidays we had together after the War. I now find I dislike the indoor, overheated modern, swimming pools with their strong chlorine and chemical smells. Changing into a swimsuit and getting wet in cold, possibly polluted seawater is almost as uninviting nowadays, although I used to love swimming in the open air. My delight in swimming seems to have vanished, unless I had my own mildly heated, open-air, large swimming pool. One can indulge in dreams!

We had a family holiday at Minehead in Somerset in the summer of 1937. My only memories of this are of having donkey rides on the beach, watching the Punch and Judy show and the sea being a long way away. The last summer holiday I spent with both my parents was when I was seven, and it is the clearest memory I have of us all together. In the summer of 1938 we stayed for a week at Gorleston-on-sea, near Lowestoft, in Suffolk. I don't know whether it was a regular custom of the period to have a kind of combined 'boarding-house and semi-self-catering' holiday, but that is how I recall we were looked after. We stayed in a terraced family residence, similar to the many small guesthouses or boarding houses found at all popular seaside resorts. I think that our breakfasts were provided, and that my mother went out shopping for food each morning for our main meals, which our landlady cooked for us each day. It seems an unusual arrangement and maybe my memory is playing tricks.

The landlady's daughter was about my own age, with the unusual name of Thirzah. She became very attached to our little family - and I became very fond of Thirzah. We wanted to go out and play on the beach together, so she accompanied my parents and me each day as we set off for the front each morning. It was a happy summer holiday, as Thirzah and I made sand pies and built castles on the beach, paddled and bathed in the sea, while the sun shone brilliantly each day. No doubt our preoccupations and pleasures enabled my mother and father to relax, snooze and read the paper in their deck chairs without having to keep me amused.

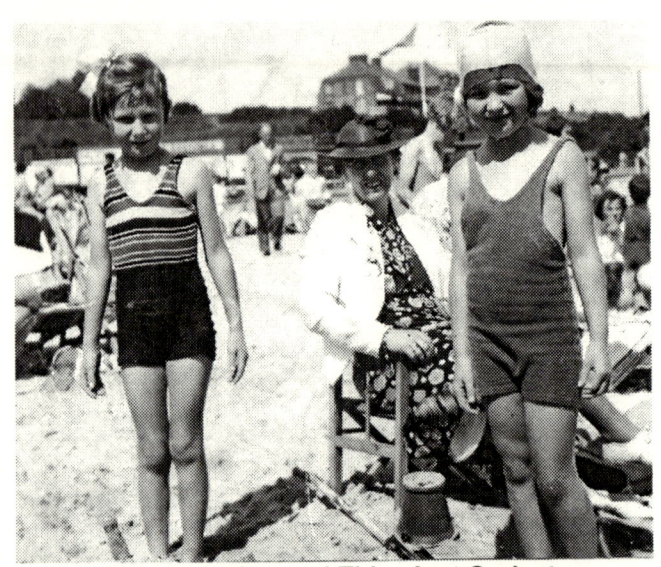

With my mother and Thirzah at Gorleston

One afternoon Thirzah and I wandered off barefoot to the pier in our swimsuits. Thirzah accidentally trod on a piece of rough wood and got a large, dirty splinter in her foot. She was in great pain and tried hard to hold back her tears as I helped her to limp painfully back to my parents, who took her to the local hospital in the car to have the splinter removed. She soon recovered sufficiently to prepare for a fancy dress party we had both been invited to on the day before I returned home. I was dressed, reluctantly, as a jester in a two-coloured outfit, with a funny, floppy hat with bells on my head. I didn't understand why I had to appear in such a peculiar outfit and I got 'cold feet' as the time approached to leave for the party. I had never been dressed up in this way before, was unfamiliar with children's parties and felt too shy to show myself off in this weird attire. I didn't understand what a jester was, or why my costume looked (to me) so odd, and I refused to go. It must have been a disappointment for Thirzah and possibly for her parents too. They may have arranged for me to be invited to the party as a little 'thank you' to my parents for taking their daughter out and about during the week. For many years there was a photo of Thirzah and me in our respective fancy dress gear in our drawer of oddments. I often used to open the drawer in the needlework cabinet, search until I found this picture and then take it out to remind myself of my brief friendship on that lovely holiday. I wonder what happened to the photo? These little reminders of the past are often thought unimportant and are thrown away.

Our holiday came to a close and parting was very painful for me. I can remember crying for a long time in the back seat of the car as we drove home, and my father told me years later that I cried all the way to Ipswich! I never heard from Thirzah again and I didn't write to her, but I often wonder what happened to my surrogate 'sister' whom I knew for only a week. Neither of us thought to write to each other. Children corresponding with or telephoning friends was not common then. I never came across the name Thirzah again, until very recently while reading a book by Sybil Marshall, which was set in East Anglia. Perhaps it is a name more common in that part of England.

Other childhood outings were occasional visits to the cinema. I remember the day I was taken to the pictures to see the 'Hunchback of Notre Dame'. I cannot imagine why I could have been taken to see this very frightening film as a small child, but I can clearly remember covering my face with my black velour school hat during many of the very scary bits, when Charles Laughton as Quasimodo clambered around Notre Dame Cathedral tower and was so cruelly treated. His distorted face, hunched back and deformed figure, and the huge bells in the dark church tower can still be recalled.

I have no bad memories concerning the occasion my parents took me to see 'Snow White and the Seven Dwarfs' in about 1938, with the delight of seeing this film in colour. I loved every moment of it, especially the memorable songs, the antics of the dwarfs and the wonderful exaggerated expressions of their eyes. I think this was not long before my mother had her next serious illness. Another early childhood visit to the 'pictures' was to see 'Sabu the Elephant Boy'. I was thrilled to watch his adventures as he grew up in the jungle. I also saw some of Shirley Temple's films and can remember her strange, high-pitched voice singing 'Animal Crackers in My Soup' and her blonde 'bubbles' hairstyle.

'Bubbles' certainly would not have been the word used to describe my own hair, which was straight, and cut short to the nape of my neck, in a style that was called a 'bob'. I sometimes had a satin hair ribbon tied in a bow on one side of my hair, plus a slide to hold it in place. The slide controlled my fair hair better than a ribbon, which often used to slip off. My mother used to tell me at teatime that 'if you eat the crusts from your bread it will make your hair curl'. It wasn't true! My parents sometimes repeated the little rhyme - 'There was a little girl and she had a little curl, right in the middle of her forehead. When she was good, she was very, very good, but when she was bad, she was horrid' - to me. I always had straight hair, so presume this ditty was recited to me when I was 'horrid'.

When I was older our housekeeper's daughter and I sometimes had our hair wound up with 'rags' before we went to bed. The 'rags' were strips of old sheeting, rather like bandages; small clumps of hair were rolled up in each 'rag', and tied securely close to our head. They were very hard, knobbly and uncomfortable to sleep in. The resultant curls or waves in my hair the next morning were not worth the discomfort of these old-fashioned 'curlers', but when Rose's simple rag curlers were unwound in the morning her hair fell naturally into long dark ringlets.

My mother had a short hairstyle with a slight wave on one side, which she produced with the aid of curling tongs. She heated these up on the gas ring of our old-fashioned stove and tested their temperature by pressing the tongs between sheets of newspaper. If the newspaper was not scorched but nicely curved and light brown, the tongs were considered to be the right temperature to put into her hair. She held them there for a short while for the heat and pressure of the iron to put in a wave. This procedure produced a wave or two in her hair and a smell of hot metal and slightly burned newspaper that I can still sense! It is strange how many memories are strengthened by the recollection of the associated smell.

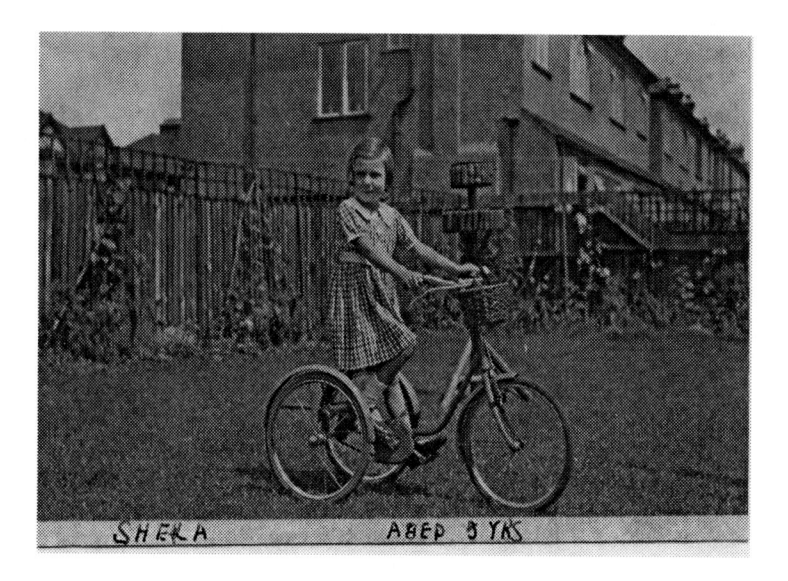

Riding my tricycle in the garden

I can recall pedalling along on my blue tricycle beside my mother as she walked the mile or so to our main shopping centre in Kenton High Street to have her hair cut, or a 'Marcel' wave in a ladies' hairdressing salon next door to our nearest Sainsbury's. Perhaps a 'Marcel' wave was similar to a hair 'set' nowadays (or was the term used then for a perm?) I cannot remember my mother with any hairstyle resembling the traditional tightly curled or permanently waved hair so common in those days. Neither have I any recollection of having my own haircut, but it must have occurred at regular intervals. Perhaps my mother cut my hair? It was always cut short until I was about twelve or thirteen, when I grew it longer (it was still straight) and I wore it tied in two 'bunches' with a ribbon at Senior School.

Sainsbury's was a long shop that went back a good distance from its entrance, (rather like my father's shop, Meakers). It was not a supermarket then, but there was a delicatessen counter, butchery, a dairy and a grocery department. Sainsbury's grocer's store did not sell toilet rolls, soap powders nor fruit and vegetables. The glass or marble-topped counters had dark polished mahogany fronts for different kinds of groceries. Customers queued at the dairy counter, where a dexterous Assistant used two wooden butter patters to cut off a lump of butter from a large block. With much skilful clicking and patting she trimmed and shaped the piece of butter to the weight asked for by the customer. Eggs were placed in a brown paper bag. Biscuits were displayed in large cube-shaped tins placed at an angle in front of the counter and the customer indicated the type of biscuit she required. The assistant then leaned forward from behind the counter and picked up a handful or two of loose biscuits from the tin, put them in a brown paper bag, placed it on the scales and weighed up the required amount (usually half-a-pound). Any extra biscuits were tossed back into the tin. I cannot conceive how customers managed to arrive home with their biscuits unbroken, let alone be able to unpack un-cracked eggs from their shopping baskets.

Another counter was specifically for 'dry' groceries – cereals, flour, sugar etc. There was also a delicatessen counter, where, among other savoury meats and pies, one could buy deliciously smelling, freshly cooked, hot Saveloy sausage. Occasionally my mother bought a piece of this and I can remember being given a small chunk of this succulent, spicy sausage, with a shiny brown skin, to eat as we made our way home.

Shopping was quite a tedious business at Sainsbury's, waiting to be served at the different counters. Payment for all food was, of course, made in cash. There were no chequebooks, no plastic cards. An imposing cash desk set in an alcove and framed by a surround of carved, dark, polished wood, was at the far end of the shop, where the cashier sat behind her till waiting to attend to the customers. The assistants at the food counters did not handle any cash.

We did not shop regularly in the main Kenton shopping centre. It was too far from home to carry all our shopping, and our local parade of shops provided us with all our daily needs. My mother only went there to get delicatessen treats - especially Saveloy sausage, as far as I was concerned - if she happened to be in the main Kenton shopping street for a hair-do. Sometimes she bought live eels from a tank of water in front of the fishmonger's shop in Kenton High Street. My mother selected which slithering fish she fancied, the fishmonger wrapped it up in newspaper and it was brought home – presumably having rapidly died, and cooked it for our dinner. I don't think that the horrible thoughts that occur to me now as I describe this even entered my head when I was a child!

As I cycled along on my tricycle by my mother's side one afternoon I was singing a popular song 'Any umbrellas, any umbrellas, to sell today' that I had heard on the wireless. Yet another tiny fragment of memory! Maybe there had been a shower of rain as we made our way home. There seemed to be so much more singing and whistling when I was young. Errand boys and boys on bicycles whistled the latest tune as they cycled passed. The popular songs that we heard on the wireless were on our lips and there was none of the overloud pop music emerging from car windows that one hears nowadays as the traffic roars by.

I remember hearing "The Lambeth Walk" on the radio one day and dancing around the dining room with my mother. I think this is one of the very few memories I have of actually doing something with my mother. The song must have been the latest hit when the show "Me and My Girl" was first performed in 1937 - top of the pops? A year or two later the War songs were on everybody's lips - "Run, rabbit, run rabbit, run, run, run", "We'll meet again, don't know where, don't know when", "The White Cliffs of Dover", and so many others that my mother probably never heard. She would have known or understood very little of the passage of the War years, and I have no idea what life must have been like for her in a Psychiatric Hospital during that period.

Long before that time came however, I was kneeling on the Put-u-Up beneath our dining room window and looking across our front garden as I watched the children going along the road to school. I longed to be among them. The usual suburban golden privet hedge divided our garden from that of our next-door neighbour's, but in the winter the colour was rather drab. My father had planted a row of irises beneath the window and another in the bed behind the little garden fence. These would produce their colourful blue 'flags' in the spring, but the spiky leaves were brown at the tips and a little dreary in wintertime. Between the front lawn and the driveway was a flower border in which my father had planted several standard roses, with clumps of what we used to call ice plant (sedum) in between.

Everything looked rather dull and lifeless in the winter of 1935 and the weather seemed wet and miserable too as I recall watching the children chatting to each other as they hurried by on their way to school. Even quite young children were unaccompanied by a parent in those days and walked or ran to school on their own or with their friends. There was very little traffic on the roads and children were able to cross Kenton Lane at the Belisha crossing situated near the road the school was in. There was no undue concern for the safety of children in our quiet suburban streets and no fear of undesirable attention or speeding cars. I knew that I would soon be joining those children and could hardly wait for my fifth birthday to occur in the summer.

The months seemed to drag by but at last my mother took me along the road and into the classroom for my first morning at school. The room seemed very large; it was probably the biggest room I had ever been in and its apparent vastness appeared a little overwhelming to a small five-year-old. There was a big dolls' house in one corner and I was attracted to this and went over to play with it while my mother was registering me with the teacher, Miss Garwood. I had been looking forward to this new event in my life, was not at all worried, and soon settled down to school routine.

School dinners were not available in those pre-war days and I came home each day for my mid-day meal, running back to school again on my own in the afternoon. There were no nursery schools or pre-school playgroups to introduce children to the process of learning or socialising. There was no preliminary visit to the school and no gradual introduction to the new realm of the classroom. We did our pre-school 'learning' at home. I had a book of nursery rhymes when I was a little girl and I liked the rhyme, the rhythm and the brief stories they expressed, but I can still remember what must have been the first little poem (if such it can be called) that I learned at Infant School. My Auntie Ada and my schoolteacher Uncle Bert were visiting my parents, and my mother persuaded me to recite ,my 'party piece'. I stood somewhat reluctantly with my back to the dining room door and rattled off the words: 'The berries on the bushes are dressing up in red. "I wonder why they do it?" a little birdie said. "I know," said Robin Redbreast, who hopped upon a tree; it helps to make them easy for little birds to see".' Why this little ditty has stayed in my mind for seventy years I cannot imagine, but I think of it every time I see 'the berries on the bushes' in winter.

The playground singing games we learned in Infant School gave me much pleasure, and I was surprised recently to hear neighbours' children playing the same games as they sang 'In and out the windows' and 'The Farmer's in his Den' in their back garden in the summertime. It is good to know that some traditions are passed on from days gone by and are still known today. (Some of the warm-up exercises we do in my present rather 'elderly' Keep Fit Class are not all that dissimilar to some of our Infant School exercise activities in the playground! Could it be our 'second childhood'?)

One year, I think it was 1938; a large Union flag was hoisted up a flagpole on Empire Day. The entire school gathered in front of the flag. It was a special ceremony when someone of some local importance addressed us all before we sang the National Anthem. I think this occurred the year before the War began. Each child was then presented with a fruit from somewhere in the British Empire. I received a very small, reddish-skinned banana, but I had no idea what country it came from and I thought it was a very strange banana. I had little understanding of the significance or vastness of the Empire or the world it was a part of, and certainly did not appreciate the great distance across the ocean that my banana had travelled. Bananas disappeared a year or two later when the dangers of enemy action at sea prevented even essential supplies from reaching our shores and our shops. Exotic fruits like bananas were never seen, and oranges were a very rare wartime treat. I am sure I greatly under-valued my Empire-Day-banana of unusual colour.

A rag-and-bone man or a gypsy occasionally stood outside the School gate at dinnertime, telling the children that if we brought back some 'rags' for him in the afternoon he would exchange them for a goldfish. I hurried home excitedly, asked my mother for some old clothes, and returned to school after my dinner with a brown paper carrier bag (no plastic bags in those days) containing some old clothing or unwanted household material. At the end of the afternoon a flurry of young children rushed out of school, all carrying our bags of rags, to see if the rag-and-bone man was at the gate with his old horse and cart. We were all eager to exchange our offerings for a watery 'pet'. As I handed over my carrier bag, he exchanged it for a tiny goldfish, which he slid into a jam jar of water. I tried not to spill any water as I carefully walked home with my hapless little fish being bumped around. My mother found a bowl to put it in and we bought some fish food from our local ironmonger's shop, but my new treasured 'pet' did not live very long. This practice would be illegal nowadays - and quite rightly so - but it provided much excitement when I was young.

I enjoyed learning to read, although I cannot remember the name of the reading scheme that was used, but I am sure that if I saw a selection of reading schemes of that period, I would recognise the series of books - about a farmer and his farm animals. Learning to read came easily to me and throughout my life I have derived much pleasure from reading. I remember very little else from my early infant school days. I have no recollection of owning any books when I was young, apart from my book of Nursery Rhymes, but clearly recall the new public Library being built quite near to our home. It was a large, ultra-modern building, somewhat in the 1930s Bauhaus style of architecture, and my mother took me to see it before it opened to the public. She lifted me up to look through the windows, where I was able to glimpse the shelves full of books in the Children's Library, and view the large, solid, light-coloured, polished wooden tables surrounded by big chairs with green leather upholstery. As soon as the Library opened my mother took me along the road to join, but I had to wait until I had reached my seventh birthday before I was allowed to have my own Library tickets. Until then my books were borrowed with my mother's ticket. When that magic age arrived I was proud, and quite awed, to be allowed to go unaccompanied into the Children's Section of the Library, choose my own books and use my own tickets. I then waited in line at the counter for the librarian, Miss Dimbleby, to date-stamp the books and remove the tickets from their little cardboard pockets.

I remember the Milly-Molly-Mandy books and although I have never heard of them or seen them since I was little, they remain vividly in my memory. I loved these books and recall a chapter in one of them about Milly-Molly-Mandy having potatoes baked in their jackets in the ashes of a bonfire. I was eager to have potatoes baked in the same way, and one Guy Fawkes Night my father made a bonfire in the back garden; my mother placed potatoes in their skins in the hot ashes, then we waited impatiently for them to cook. I can only recall this one celebration of Guy Fawkes, and picture only the sparklers and the bonfire, but I can still savour the taste and smell of the potatoes, sprinkled with salt and a blob of fresh butter to add to the special taste of wood-ash-baked potatoes.

When I was a little older I lapped up the "Just William" books, "Dr. Doolittle" series, and "The Swallows and Amazons". Later on I was hooked on schoolgirl-stories. No horror stories, or stories about schoolgirl sex, single teenage mothers, or broken homes in those days, just harmless, amusing reading matter, with well-constructed sentences which filled the mind with the imaginary life of girls' boarding schools, 'dorms', crushes, hockey matches and other childish adventures.

The Library was to become almost a second home to me in the winter during school holidays in the War. It was warm and comfortable and I could sit and read to my heart's content on the green leather chairs. When fuel shortages prevented a fire being lit at home until teatime, it was often cosier to sit in the Library during the day. It always had a quiet atmosphere, with any conversation exchanged in a whisper. I am sure my enjoyment of reading was much encouraged by this excellent County Library. It is still there, looking much as it did in the l930s, on the corner of what is now a fairly busy cross-roads with traffic lights; no longer the quiet suburban streets of the mid-nineteen-thirties.

I don't know whether my parents made much use of the Library when it first opened. I think they were busy laying out the garden when my mother was well, but they may have relaxed with a Library book in the winter evenings, as well as listening to the wireless after I had gone to bed. My mother browsed among the books in the Adult Library while I was selecting my books in the Junior Section when the Library first opened, so she probably enjoyed reading. I know my father borrowed books regularly. There was no TV entertainment for anybody during the War and apart from reading; the 'wireless' set was the main form of recreation in our house.

I had the opportunity of seeing television one afternoon before the War began. I was invited to tea with a girl who lived nearby. We shared the same Christian name and I think this was the only time I went into her house. Maybe the invitation was to show off this revolutionary piece of equipment. After tea the curtains were drawn and Sheila, her two sisters, Valerie and Vivienne and I sprawled on the floor, chins cupped in our hands and elbows propped up on the carpet in the darkened room. Our eyes were fixed on the square of flickering grey pictures moving on a small glass screen. The television cabinet was very big and cumbersome and seemed to dominate the room. I was unable to comprehend what the film was about; the picture was fuzzy and the speech indistinct. I much preferred listening to Children's Hour on the wireless with 'Uncle David' and 'Uncle Mac' telling stories, the serial 'Toytown' and the story of 'Black Beauty'.

Chapter Five

CHILDHOOD TOYS AND PASTIMES

I can remember only three toys from my early years at Osterley. I treasured a red box with a small 'golden' metal hook and clip that made the box itself seem precious and intriguing to me. Twelve wooden cubes were inside, with part of a picture of a farm animal stuck on each side. A complete picture of one of the six animals gradually appeared as I turned the blocks to the correct position, but the metal hook and clip on this special red wooden box were as interesting to me as the puzzle inside it. Another favourite toy was a set of coloured building blocks - rectangles, cubes, triangles, curved arches and pillars. Two of these blocks were the ones stuck on to our kitchen window-ledge some years later, to support the clock from my father's old Austin 7 car. Together with the pedal car, which frustrated my youthful desires for speedy driving, these are the only toys I remember from my first home.

Having friends to tea were very rare occasions in my childhood. In fact I can only remember one occasion when my mother was at home in which I had some friends to tea. I think this was on my birthday in 1936. I have an old snapshot of three little girls sitting sedately in the back garden with our arms folded, hair neatly combed, wearing summer dresses and white ankle socks. A little boy is standing stalwartly behind us – Johnny Boughton – in his position as the only male. It must have been a very decorous, well-behaved little affair. I can remember nothing of the games we may have played or the tea we ate, or of my mother's organisation of this little party for my fifth birthday.

My parents gave me a splendid, modern, flat-roofed doll's house for Christmas following our move to Kenton. It had white painted walls just like the outside of our new home. Battery-powered electricity enabled me to light up each of the rooms. I recall that the battery (neatly positioned on the flat roof) ran down rather quickly, probably because I sometimes left the switch on. The dolls' house was kept in my bedroom, and I enjoyed playing with my small 'property' with its' sets of miniature furniture given to me by my Auntie Ada from time to time.

I also had a beautiful, flaxen-haired china doll, with blue eyes, long eyelashes and eyelids that opened and closed. She said 'ma-ma' when her tummy was pressed. An old snap-shot shows me standing beneath one of the rustic arches in our new garden, proudly nursing my shawl-wrapped doll. I had named her Audrey after a little girl I occasionally played with when staying with my Auntie Ada. Audrey's little pram – or bassinet, as my Aunt called it - was kept in our hall. Like most little girls, I played with my doll, but although I was fond of her, she never totally absorbed my attention. I didn't quite know what to do with this beautiful 'baby' once she had been dressed and laid in her little pram. I enjoyed wheeling the perambulator when going to the shops with my mother each day, with Audrey proudly propped up against her little pillow. Before every household had a refrigerator, shopping was an important part of the daily round of a housewife's life.

One day a major tragedy occurred in my small world. My mother and I went on a shopping expedition that required a bus ride to Harrow. We were going to 'Sopers', a large department store now owned by Debenham's, so Audrey and her pram were left at home. I sat her up in one of the old brown leather armchairs in the dining room before we set off. Betty, our Airedale puppy, had also been left behind, lying asleep on the dining room floor. She was growing into a large dog, getting frisky, and would not be allowed on the bus. When we returned from our shopping trip we found small pieces of white plaster-of-Paris and dust all over the room. The furniture was smothered with white powder and Audrey was almost non-existent. Betty had woken up, got bored and fractious and decided that my beloved doll was her plaything to be tussled and tugged. Perhaps she was jealous of this perceived rival; she had chewed and mauled my precious doll to pieces, almost nothing but dust remained of her - literally, dust to dust! I was heartbroken and almost inconsolable at my loss. Perhaps I loved her more in her 'death' than I did in her 'life'. My Auntie Ada gave me another doll to replace her, whom I also named Audrey, but she never replaced Audrey-number-one in my affection.

My mother sometimes gave me a jam-jar full of soapsuds when she was doing the washing on a Monday morning. I would spend a contented half hour in the garden blowing colourful translucent soap bubbles into the air from a little clay bubble-pipe, watching them gradually rise up towards the sky before they burst. I had a wooden hoop and sometimes bowled it along with my hand down the garden path beside our garage, or into the sideway. Another way of passing the time was to stand by our front gates with a paper and pencil, waiting for a car to drive along the road, to hastily note down the car number. Cars were not frequently seen even in our wide suburban street, and collecting car numbers was a pleasant but rather unexciting pastime on a sunny day. I wasn't at all interested in the names of the different makes of cars. This was a boy's hobby and would certainly have absorbed my husband's attention. Only the registration numbers were written down on my little list.

I kept my toys in the bottom of one of the fitted cupboards in my bedroom. I had a number of colouring and painting books and remember spending wet afternoons sitting at the enamel-topped kitchen table with a jam-jar of water, dabbing my paint-brush over the pages of a 'magic' painting book. As one dampened each page with the wet brush a colourful picture emerged on the paper, filling in the printed outline and miraculously producing a complete scene. There was not a lot of creativity in this occupation! Puzzle books, with dot-to-dot pictures, mazes and other pencil and paper games whiled away many hours. I don't ever remember doing free-hand painting or drawing.

A little printing set containing different rubber printing blocks with the outline of a postman, a tree, a ship and other figures, made another indoor activity. I pressed each small wooden backed block into an inkpad, then on to a sheet of paper and produced black outlines of these little objects. I completed the printing process by setting a line of tiny rubber letters into another little block and printed titles to accompany my rather smudgy printed pictures. This was all very laborious and very messy, as I recall.

Another pastime was called 'French knitting'. My father banged four nails into the top of an empty cotton reel and then I pushed the end of a small ball of wool through the hole in the middle of the reel. The wool was wound twice round the nails before I could begin the 'knitting', hooking the lower loop of wool over each nail with a small crochet hook (when did I last see a crochet hook?), to form a knot or stitch. The 'knitting' worked its way through the middle of the reel as I continued winding the wool around the nails and hooking the wool over them. A tube of coloured 'knitting' eventually appeared at the other end of the cotton reel, gradually lengthened until it was long enough for me to sew the long thin 'sausage' of knitting round and round into a little mat. I am not at all sure what happened to the finished product. Sewing pictures on cards with holes pricked in them at regular intervals was yet another activity. After I had stitched my coloured wool through the appropriate holes the outline of a simple picture appeared.

A pack of Happy Families cards entertained many children in those days. The pictures of the Butcher's family, the Baker's family the other families in this children's card game interested me. I must have played this game with my parents or with friends but I can only recall sitting at the dining table on my own, sorting out the pictures into their different 'Families'. I also had Ludo and Snakes and Ladders. I remember playing these board games, but cannot visualise with whom I played at home, although I remember playing similar games at a friend's house when I was a little older. I don't ever remember other children coming to the house to play.

My Aunt once took me to see Father Christmas in his 'Grotto' in a big store in Lewisham. He gave me a present of a box of different-coloured small balls in a cardboard tray full of holes, and I subsequently spent many happy hours sitting on my bedroom floor arranging these balls into a variety of mosaic patterns. It was a well remembered and much used present from a friendly, non-frightening 'Father Christmas'.

All these games and toys seem so simple and were not very creative, educative or stimulating when compared with the vast array of toys that children have nowadays. As I describe my childhood occupations I realise that we were a very undemanding generation of children, whose expectations were not high. Especially designed educational and child-development toys did not exist. Special children's books were not common possessions in the homes of ordinary folk, although I do remember looking at my cousin Daphne's wonderful 'pop-up' picture books when staying with my Auntie Lily. Daphne was six years older than I and had outgrown these books, which would have been published before the War began. I was thrilled to see the 'hidden' pictures appear as I slowly turned the pages of her magical books. The inside of a tree trunk was revealed when I pulled the tabs on some pages, when all the insects and little creatures that lived in the tree suddenly became visible. On another page the birds that nested in the branches appeared in an instant. Yet other pages were covered with coloured cellophane that mysteriously changed the character of the picture, and still further mysteries unfolded when cut-out pictures suddenly popped up as I turned to them. I was fascinated by these books; they gave me much delight and remain in my memory. I had none of these elaborate and fancy books of my own. No doubt wartime restrictions and paper shortages from 1939 onwards had an effect on the availability of children's books, prohibiting any intricate or quality printing.

My parents gave me a blue tricycle for Christmas soon after I started school in 1936. They had managed to carry the tricycle upstairs after I had gone to bed on Christmas Eve and I found it when I went into their bedroom early on Christmas morning. I was so excited, and especially loved the bell and the little shopping basket on the handlebars. My mother sat on the saddle in the bedroom, moving the handlebars to left and right and ringing the little bell, but I remember being worried that she looked a bit too large to sit on the saddle of my new acquisition! I knew this present did not come from Father Christmas and that it was a gift from my parents. I don't know how or why it was brought upstairs. Their bedroom had a fireplace, so perhaps it was placed there because of my earlier fear of Santa coming through my bedroom window in an airplane - but by then I knew he wasn't real!

I find it strange that I cannot remember ever having a Christmas stocking. Maybe I did have one, but because I knew that it did not appear mysteriously as a gift from Father Christmas it has not remained in my memory at all. Although the country was in the midst of the Economic Depression of the Thirties, it did not seem to have affected my father's business and I think I was lucky enough to have 'real' presents. A stocking was perhaps considered to be a relic of earlier, poorer days. My father told me that when he was young he had to be content with an orange, a penny, a pencil, a sugary sweet and a simple home-made toy in a sock for Christmas, if he was lucky. (Christmas stockings became a tradition after I married and had my own children. I am sure I gained as much pleasure over finding intriguing little presents and stuffing their stockings to the brim, as they did on waking in the early hours of Christmas morning, and searching for their gifts from 'Father Christmas', even after they knew where these little surprise presents came from. Their 'real' gifts came a little later in the Day.)

After I started school I began to learn the playground games that most children enjoyed. Skipping was always a favourite pastime with the girls, and the skipping games, rhymes and movements became more complicated as we grew older. A long rope was held during the skipping 'season' at Junior School and turned vigorously by a girl at either end. First one, then a second and a third girl jumped into the swiftly arching rope. Eventually someone tripped up, mistimed their entry, or caught a toe in the rope and stopped the combined jumping. Playtimes passed quickly and happily as we skipped with our own shorter ropes and intoned the old skipping rhymes... 'I like coffee, I like tea, I like (name of a friend) in with me', whereupon the named friend smartly joined in the jump as the rope turned again. 'Salt, mustard, vinegar, pepper' was another rhyme, with a jump on the turn for each word and a double turn and jump on the word 'pepper'. We called these fast double turns in time with a jump: 'bumps'. 'A house to rent, no rent to pay, knock at the door, and run away' was yet another skipping rhyme with a 'bump' to emphasise the last word of each line.

We spent many 'playtime' hours with these energetic skipping games and then running/skipping home along the pavement after school was over. In the light of present-day advice that foot-pounding exercise is good for the heart, keeps the weight down and helps to prevent osteoporosis, we must have done a lot in those days to reduce the likelihood of developing these conditions in our later years! Our healthy, outdoor, aerobic exercise made our bones strong and no doubt strengthened the function of our hearts. These playground games also taught us good co-ordination, rhythm and how to interact in a group activity. What fun we had with our skipping ropes - which were often just lengths of spare washing line.

Our games were seasonal. At another time of the year we all suddenly, it seemed, started playing marbles. I had a good collection of coloured glass marbles that I kept in a little cloth bag. Two people played together; the first rolled her marble a little way along the playground, or the gutter if we were playing on our way home from school. (There was no traffic to worry about and roads, gutters and pavements were well maintained by Harrow Urban District Council and regularly swept by the road-sweeper - a man with a long, stiff broom and a little handcart. Streets, pavements and gutters were much cleaner than nowadays). Then the second player aimed her marble carefully at her opponent's. If she hit it, the marble was hers, but if she didn't, the first person aimed her marble at the second one, until one or the other won. I had a good eye for marbles, aimed carefully and hoarded quite a collection of colourful winnings, frequently examining them for their individual characteristics and beauty! We also treasured some very special, big marbles, that we called 'Queenies'. I am not sure of their particular purpose, but they were very collectable. I sometimes purchased one of these special marbles with my weekly pocket money after much pondering over which one was the best value or most beautiful.

'Five stones' was another craze that occurred annually. Each player found five small, smooth pebbles, and a little group of friends crouched close to the playground tarmac. We took it in turn to hold all the stones in the palm of our hand before throwing them in the air and trying to catch one on the back of the hand. The game continued with complicated arranging and catching of groups of two, three and four stones without dropping one, until five were caught in the palm of the hand. It was quite a skilful, complicated and lengthy game. 'Five stones' season usually occurred during the summer months when the weather was too hot for more active games.

We played hopscotch, not with a painted plan of the game provided for us by funds from a School PTA (unheard of), but one that we marked out with a piece of chalk or a sharp broken stone on the playground or the pavement. Then we commenced our game by throwing a stone into square number one and jumping through the set pattern. Our games were not costly. Handstands were another craze in the summer, when our cotton frocks were in great disarray, but one that I didn't enjoy very much. I have never liked having my head upside-down. Many primary school playgrounds today are well covered with outlines of games, lots of equipment, and ideas for various activities that did not exist even when my own children were at school over forty years ago. We all had to invent our own outdoor amusements.

A small rubber ball or an old tennis ball provided a wide range of games that developed our ball handling skills. I always enjoyed ball games, even if it was only bouncing a ball against a brick wall (the wartime brick air raid shelters in the nearby side street where my friend Joan lived were ideal!), throwing and catching it in different ways. One could play on one's own, or take it in turns with a friend, throwing the ball over-arm, under-arm, bounce it on the ground on the way to the wall, then letting it bounce on its return before catching it. We threw it to the wall from around our back, we caught the ball after clapping our hands, throwing and catching with one hand, then the other, then bounced it towards the wall by throwing it between our legs, then under one raised leg, or the other. The variations were almost endless. Once a 'catch' had been missed, your 'turn' was over. As we grew older and were allowed to stay up longer and go out after tea, my friend Joan and I spent the long summer evenings playing ball in the street. Sometimes we stood in the middle of the narrow road in which Joan lived, throwing the ball to each other high in the air over the telegraph wires. It made us into good 'fielders' in rounders in Secondary School years with our well-developed over-arm throw! It also provided us with much pleasure, exercise, fresh air and comradeship at the time. I am sure my ability to be able to play tennis until my early seventies owed much to the simple ball skills I developed when I was young; getting 'my eye in' and developing stamina.

I wonder how many children play the old traditional games today. Although they are being encouraged to be more physically active in schools now, I suspect many prefer to spend their spare time indoors watching TV, playing video games, working their computer, surfing the Internet, on their mobile phones, texting, considering their clothes, make-up, magazines, weight, boy/girl friends, hairstyle etc. - or going to the Health and Fitness Club with their parents. We thought nothing of these things; most of them did not exist; others, like fashionable, trendy or casual clothes, were unobtainable. There was little provision of organised clubs and activities or parental involvement in children's leisure activities; we developed our own hobbies and games, and the streets were safe to play in.

We had no interest in make-up in Junior School or Secondary School, and sex did not appear on our horizons for many years. We were also burdened with much less homework and school projects than young people are given today. We were considered children until we were into our teens, although a high degree of good (and mature) behaviour was expected of us. School-leavers were very unsophisticated when they were suddenly transferred into the adult working world at fourteen or sixteen years of age. The terms 'teens' and 'teenager' are comparatively new words in the English vocabulary and would not have appeared in any dictionary when I was at school. Similarly, none of the modern computer-age language or text-messages had as yet been dreamed of, but we did learn to spell and use the English language correctly and speak it clearly! We didn't 'grunt'! Very few of the vulgar slang and swear words that are so commonly heard today, and used so freely by many in everyday speech, were even known by us. They were certainly not spoken on the radio or in school, heard in my home, or in day-to-day conversation with friends. I don't remember anyone at my Primary School and very few at my Secondary School, blaspheming, swearing, or using obscene or vulgar language. We lived in a different world, a more wholesome, respectful and God-fearing one I think, and yet, a more insular one.

We were oblivious of the existence of famine, drought, poverty or a 'Third World'. Most of us were totally ignorant about the existence of the disadvantaged in other parts of our own country or of the restrictions of the disabled kept hidden in their own homes or institutions. Those who were mentally ill or mentally handicapped were shut away and were largely ignored, mocked or despised by society, unless one had a member of one's own family in some way afflicted - then you kept very quiet about it. We understood little about the progress of the War. However, we became a little more informed of the needs of others when the War ended - of the homeless, the starving, the refugees, or those who had suffered, lost loved ones or managed to survive in the concentration camps. Although we were well aware of the War's immediate effects on our lives – shortages, ration books for food and clothing, air raids etc. - we had no knowledge of global issues, or fear of sudden political uprisings or international terrorism. Newspapers were quite small, with a few grainy, black and white pictures. There was little reporting of sports, usually printed on the back page, or reviews of books, plays etc., and almost no fashion, health or beauty articles. There were no glossy weekend supplements and whole page advertisements that appear in today's massive newspapers, which use up so much of the world's natural resources. It was many years before television became available to most of the population, giving pictures and information about what was happening in all parts of the globe. Our interests and pastimes were largely homemade!

Chapter Six

GREAT CHANGES

My father had opened his own men's outfitters' shop in the early l930s at Southall, in Middlesex. In those days Southall was part of suburbia on the fringe of London, but it is now absorbed into Greater London and has one of the largest Asian populations in the country. He employed a Manager of his new enterprise, but retained his own job as the Manager of Meakers at Ealing Broadway. Mr. Wookey and his wife soon became friends with my parents, and I remember his very pleasant West Country dialect. My blue tricycle was passed on to their daughter Josephine when it became too small for me, but sadly my father lost touch with the family after Mr. Wookey was called up into the RAF. My father saw little of his and my mother's old friends once the War started. His own reserved nature also promoted a partial withdrawal from social life, partly, I suspect, as a result of the unspoken shame of mental illness. Long-standing 'writer's cramp' meant that he had to use his left hand for writing, and correspondence was quite an ordeal for him. Exchange of Christmas cards was his only contact with a few old friends, but writing these cards was a task that he found very trying. How much easier it would have been for him to keep in touch with friends if we had been on the telephone in those days. Personal phone calls at work were only permissible in an emergency. Today's easy means of communication were not available to most ordinary folk in the first half of the twentieth century. The telephone was not installed in very many homes. There were no slogans telling the public that 'it is good to talk'; the explosion of mobile 'phones, Fax, E-mail, the Internet and its associated technology was not yet in the realm of science fiction.

Anxiety during the period leading up to the outbreak of the War in 1939 may have contributed to, or triggered, the complete nervous breakdown my mother had in the summer of that year, combined, perhaps, with worry over my father's business venture. I now realise that she was probably unwell for some while before her final admission to a Mental Hospital in the summer of 1939. Prior to this I sometimes came home from school and found her sitting in a chair in the kitchen with her head in her hands, rocking from side to side, saying she was having 'one of her dizzy turns'. Maybe she was suffering from the side effects of some early drug such as lithium to try and help her condition, or was in some form of mental distress that I didn't understand when I was young. I certainly had no idea of any problem, but have remembered the 'dizzy turns'. It is possible that being alone in the house throughout the day while I was at school disturbed or depressed her.

It may have been suggested that my father should take my mother out occasionally in the evening. There were no baby-sitting circles in those days, but I can remember my parents once attempting to have an evening visit to the cinema. I had gone to bed and was presumed to be asleep, but I think I had suspected that they were planning to go out. When I heard the front door shutting quietly, I tumbled out of bed, flew downstairs, banging on the inside of the front door, crying at the letterbox, and sobbing, 'Don't leave me, don't leave me'. My parents heard my cries and came back indoors. I think my father was distraught with worry - what to do for the best for his unwell wife and how to cope with his upset daughter. They abandoned their attempted visit to the 'pictures' and their evening was spoilt.

I also have memories of my father giving my mother a glass of Guinness every evening, telling her that it was 'good for her nerves'. I seem to remember him standing over her as she drank it, and somehow I don't think she enjoyed it! At the time I am sure these little incidents were not seen by me as abnormal. My father also drove home from Ealing for lunch every day during this unsettled and worrying period for him, at the modest speed available to an early 1930s' Ford Eight car, in order to be with my mother for a short period during the middle of the day.

Many years later I learned she was having delusions about my father's behaviour and thought that he had been seeing other women in his lunch break! He came home to assure her of his constancy, but this journey did not leave him much time in which to eat his dinner. He also told me years later that he wanted to reassure himself that I was given a proper meal, as apparently my mother was not feeding me properly. I remember her bringing our dinner plates in from the kitchen to the dining room one day. There was a lamb chop on my father's plate and another on my mother's plate, but nothing on my plate. I can't remember anything about the vegetables! My father asked her why I had not been given any meat. My mother replied that I could have the 'tail ends' of their chops. The little day-to-day occurrences that may have indicated that my mother was not well did not appear odd to me at the time.

I don't think I noticed that I was not being given enough to eat, although some months later the housekeeper my father eventually employed took me to the doctor because she was concerned about my weight and thought I had 'worms' because my ribs were sticking out! I was prescribed tablespoonfuls of cod-liver-oil-and-malt each day, but as far as I can recall no unwanted residents were discovered. It was easy medicine and I thoroughly enjoyed my daily spoonfuls of the thick toffee-like mixture.

I am sure I always had a good appetite. I doubt whether many schoolgirls dieted during those years. We all tucked in whenever there was the opportunity and had never heard the term 'slimming'. Families sat down at the dining table together at mealtimes and children were expected to eat what was put in front of them. They had breakfast before they went to school and most ate a plain cooked meal when they came home at midday. Tea was usually a bread and butter meal with perhaps 'high tea' as a special treat. There were no fast-food shops to buy snacks from.

My next recollection of that summer brings me back to the beginning of my story, when I had hurriedly walked down the street in the early hours of the morning hand in hand with my father, to be 'minded' by a neighbour. Mrs. Rolph lived in a flat on the first floor of a house similar to our own. A little later in the morning I went to school as usual, crossing the main road at the Belisha beacon with her son, David, who was in my class at Priestmead School. We were sitting in the School Hall for our morning Assembly and I couldn't find a handkerchief. I whispered to David, who was sitting cross-legged on the floor beside me, that I needed to blow my nose and asked him if I could borrow his handkerchief. I used to have very frequent catarrhal colds but I don't think I had been crying. My recollection of that morning is that my emergency requirement was due to the sniffles, but maybe I was upset by the events that had occurred earlier. I am sure that although I was possibly bewildered, I did not understand that my mother had been taken out of my life. David pulled his (clean?) handkerchief from his trouser pocket and passed it to me. The need to blow my nose is my only memory of any possible distress. Were my teachers told about the emergency? I think not.

David's mother was often at our house and I believe she had befriended my mother and kept a kindly eye on her, as her last mental breakdown developed. He had an older sister named Irene who sometimes did a little shopping for my mother. David's father was a bus driver and the family seemed quite poor; there were no carpets on the floors, just the bare floorboards, and very little furniture. I went back to David's home after school was over. Irene, David and I were given our tea in, what in our home was the spare bedroom over the hall, but in this house it was Mrs. Rolph's kitchen. We ate either bread and jam, or bread and margarine, but not both margarine and jam. After tea, David and I went into the garden to play, but it was not at all like my own back garden. There were no flowerbeds or lawn, only some rough grass and a patch of bare earth. We amused ourselves making mud pies in a corner of this barren garden until my father called in the evening to take me home to an empty house. My mother had gone. I wonder now how I reacted to these sudden removals of my mother from my life. I remember no distress or upset. I must have thought that this was normal childhood.

My father had to arrange for obliging neighbours to care for me each day until he came home from work. Mr. and Mrs. Reynolds had moved. We were not close friends with our other neighbours and did not visit each other's homes. In those days 'an Englishman's home was his castle' and privacy was paramount - at any rate in my road in the suburban South East of England. Without the aid of a telephone I presume my father had to knock on neighbours' doors to ask someone to take care of me before and after school; perhaps they rallied round and offered to help. I have no idea how he managed at home, what we ate, if he was able to cook our meals, or what I did to help. Men were not at all domesticated before 'New Man' was invented. I have no recollection of our way of life together before the summer holidays began.

For some weeks David's mother and various neighbours looked after me before and after school each day. (A single lady lived on one side of us, with, I believe, her brother. I can remember going into their house with my mother before she became ill again and we were shown the budgerigars and canaries that were kept in the big front bedroom. There was no furniture in the room at all, or any curtains, and the door was quickly shut behind us to prevent the birds from escaping. The floorboards clattered beneath our feet, while the birds flew freely around the room. I disliked it intensely and I don't think Miss Kirby was ever asked to 'mind' me after school!)

A Scottish family with very strong Glaswegian accents lived on the other side, and I sometimes went to Mr. and Mrs. Grant's house until my father returned from work. I found it difficult to understand what they were saying as I had never met any other Scottish people. However, there was a close, happy, family atmosphere in their home. There were three children in the family. I played with Roy, who was about my age, and his sister Olive, who was a little older, and there was another, much older, brother. This was the largest family group I had ever been amongst. We had kippers for tea one day and Mr. Grant said he liked jam on his kippers. I never discovered whether this was a joke, a Scottish custom, or a personal fad.

My mother used to have a 'charlady' (as a home-help or cleaning lady was called then) once a week to help her with the housework, who looked after me on Saturdays at her home while my father was at work. I can still picture this lady, who had very crooked front teeth. I can mentally recall her voice and remember where she lived, but her name completely escapes my memory; yet I knew her so well. She took me on a long bus ride to Josephine Wookey's (the daughter of the Manager of my father's shop) birthday party one Saturday. We went up a staircase into a flat and I sat at a table eating jelly with a number of children whom I did not know at all. I can't remember what else we had for tea, or what games we played. I felt very ill at ease and did not enjoy the party, but all these kind people were trying to help in our family crisis.

As soon as the school term ended my father took me to live with my Auntie Ada and Uncle Bert once again. My Uncle's school holiday had also begun, so he was at home during the day, and his unmarried brother was now living with them. Uncle Viv slept in the large back bedroom that I had occupied while staying with my Aunt previously, so I now slept on a little camp bed in the smaller front room over the hall. This was my Uncle's study. His school papers, marking pens, a revolving date and month calendar and a gold propelling pencil were neatly arranged on the top of his desk. I was fascinated by the smart calendar and used to turn the little knob and watch the ivory rectangle with the day and date embossed upon it flip over to reveal the next one. I probably left my uncle a little confused as to the correct date, as the action of this calendar and the click of the slivers of ivory were of more interest to me than its accuracy. I am sure that I left it with the wrong date showing from time to time, but he was not at his desk very often in the school holiday and didn't seem to mind - or even notice.

Soon after I arrived at Beckenham there was a Carnival procession to the local park at the start of the August Bank Holiday weekend. The procession passed down Rectory Road right in front of my Aunt's house on the Saturday afternoon, and we were able to enjoy a grandstand view from the upstairs bedroom window. (We didn't stand outside on the pavement, which would have been much more exciting, and we certainly didn't go to the fun-fair in the Park!)

After I had been sent to bed that evening I decided that I wanted to record the happenings of the day. I was tempted to pick up and use my Uncle's beautiful gold propelling pencil with the red lead that he used for marking his pupils' schoolwork. I found a piece of paper, sat at my Uncle's desk, and commenced to record my 'diary' of the day's events. As I grew absorbed in my writing I made some little sound or movement that was heard by sharp adult ears downstairs and my Aunt came up to see what I was getting up to. She began to scold me for getting out of bed and using my Uncle's materials. He soon followed her upstairs to find out what all the fuss was about. My Uncle picked up my piece of writing, looked at my red print on the sheet of his school paper and apparently was impressed that his eight-year-old niece had recorded the day's events so well. I remember that he was particularly pleased that I had spelled the word 'Saturday' correctly. I was soon commended instead of being reproved. Uncle Bert also kindly said something to the effect that he thought I had done well to have learned to use a *'u'*, when the sound of the word could have led me to write it with an *'e'*. I was delighted with my bright red script but even more proud of my Uncle's approval of my spelling.

His brother Viv was more interested in gardening than spelling and I often walked down the garden path to watch him at work in the vegetable plot at the bottom of the garden. We sometimes sat and chatted amongst the neatly arranged gardening tools and different sized pots in the shed. One sunny morning I helped him plant some beetroot seeds, and

Uncle Viv showed me how to plant them correctly. He carefully turned each seed around between his fingers, pointing out to me that it must be planted a certain way to make sure the roots grew down and the plant grew up towards the light. He invited me to help him plant the seeds. I took all this seed-planting instruction seriously and examined each seed meticulously before popping it into the ground. I made sure that I placed the most pointed part of the seed downwards to encourage the root to grow down into the soil and the leaves to grow up towards the light. It was some time before I realised that there was a twinkle in Uncle Viv's eye as he watched me and that I was having my leg pulled. He was another 'teaser'!

One Wednesday afternoon my father brought my scooter with him in the car when he came to visit. I was now able to amuse myself by scooting around the crazy paving at the back of the house and then along the path down the garden and back, before whizzing round the side of the house to the front garden and up the little path to the sundial in the middle of the front lawn. After a while I was allowed to go along the pavement and sometimes ventured around the 'block'. I enjoyed this freedom, although I was forbidden to cross any roads. Rectory Road was a very long road, so scooting into unknown territory near the Railway line and exploring the adjoining streets in the long, hot, summer mornings was quite an adventure. It must have got me out of my Aunt's way for a little while too, enabling her to get on with her household duties.

My Auntie Ada, and I believe my mother, used to make 'spotted Dick' to accompany roast beef, instead of the more usual Yorkshire pudding, but I have more vivid memories of eating this in my Aunt's house than in my own home. I used to watch her making this currant suet pudding, before laying the sausage-shaped dough on a floured cloth, tying the ends and placing it in a saucepan of boiling water to cook. My aunt then served a slice of the currant-filled pudding as an accompaniment to our roast beef and vegetables; it was delicious with the gravy. I have no idea where this custom originated. Tinned peaches and evaporated milk seem in my memory to be a frequent second course.

We sometimes went for a drive in the afternoon after my Aunt had had a rest after dinner. Uncle Bert always wore a pair of leather driving gloves with large gauntlets when he was driving. Even in hot summer weather he insisted on wearing these thick gloves when he had his hands on the wheel of his car. I believe they were a nostalgic reminder for him of earlier days when he had driven an open, drop-head Alvis tourer. This was quite a fast motorcar for its time. His wife had apparently disapproved of this racy car. My father told me that my Uncle always regretted that he had succumbed to my Aunt's fear of being a passenger in this characterful car and disliked the breeze spoiling her hairdo as he drove too fast (!) along the roads. He wished he had not sold it and replaced it with the sedate black Ford Eight car they owned when I lived with them, which was similar to my father's. Quite a contrast to a drop-head Alvis!

Two sisters who lived nearby were invited to join us on one or two of these afternoon outings. We three little girls sat in the back of the car in our clean cotton summer dresses, with our cream panama hats on our heads, while Auntie Ada sat in the front with her straw hat secured to her hair-do with a hat pin and my Uncle wore a jaunty flat-topped cap. On one occasion we saw the Eldorado ice-cream man pedalling along on a kingsize tricycle carrying his stock in a large cool-box mounted in front. Uncle Bert stopped the car and my Aunt bought each of us an ice. They were the most delicious strawberry and almond flavoured ice creams I had ever tasted. Each little block of the delicately coloured pink strawberry and green Neapolitan ice creams was carefully wrapped in greaseproof paper. I licked mine very slowly and made it last a long time. Audrey (after whom I had named my long-lamented doll) and her sister ate theirs up rapidly. When we arrived home my Aunt told me that I should eat my ice cream more quickly on any future outings in case the other girls thought I had been given a larger ice. I had thought good things were made to last. Walls ice cream men with similar huge blue tricycles and dark blue refrigerated carriers containing their selection of ices, were also familiar sights in those days. They cycled around residential areas at weekends, ringing their bells to announce their presence - a welcome sound on a hot day in summer, when an ice cream was a rare treat.

I was sometimes invited to go along the road to play with these two girls in their very large garden. A large soft-fruit-growing area extended across the bottom of both their neighbours' gardens, making the garden into a T-shape. This extensive garden was a wonderfully large space for playing hide-and-seek. In the dry summer weather two of us hid on the dusty, dry soil under the old spreading blackcurrant and gooseberry bushes, while the third counted to one hundred before she began to search for us. The smell of blackcurrant bushes always reminds me of these games of so long ago.

The days tended to drag by slowly when I was indoors, especially while my Aunt had her afternoon nap. I sometimes sat in one of the deep, softly cushioned armchairs in the 'drawing room', whiling away the time by squeezing the little lavender bags that were tucked into the corners of the chairs and sniffing the perfume of the lavender. My Aunt made these little bags each autumn with the lavender flowers she picked from the garden and dried. She sometimes brought out a large box of fancy clothes with chiffon shawls, old evening dresses and other odds and ends of things for me to play with and I loved to delve deep into the box and dress up in some of her exotic clothes.

She also had a set of colourfully painted wooden eggs, which sat on the mantelpiece in her dining room. Each egg fitted perfectly inside the next and I was fascinated with them and loved to unscrew each egg to find the slightly smaller one nesting inside, and another inside that. Eventually I reached the tiniest, solid, blue egg in the very middle. They were rather like – but not nearly as beautiful as - the Russian 'dollies' or Matryushkas that we often see nowadays. These eggs were treasures to me when I was young and I was so sad that my Aunt gave them away to a charity shop shortly before she died, not realising that even as an adult, I would have loved to have owned this little remembrance of my childhood days with her.

Towards the end of August my Aunt and Uncle took me away with them on their annual holiday to Bournemouth. I guess I enjoyed bathing (was I still wearing the hand-knitted, diagonally-striped bathing costume?? - I do hope not!), playing on the sands and building castles with the help of my Uncle Bert. But my only real memory of this holiday is of writing a picture postcard to my father, telling him that I was enjoying myself and that 'the sea was still wet'. These words must have been at my Uncle's suggestion and were meant to be a little joke. I can still picture myself sitting in our boarding house bedroom, supervised by my Uncle, as I painstakingly wrote the card to my father in my best handwriting. I don't think that I even thought wistfully of him at home all alone. I just didn't understand what was happening. It is really the only memory I have of this holiday.

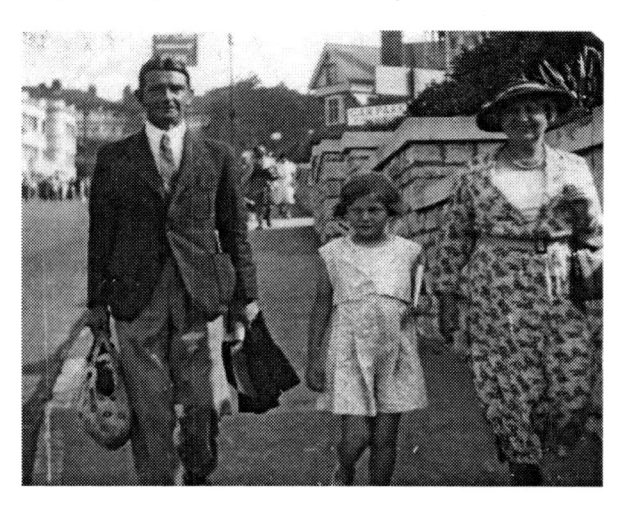

At Bournemouth with my Aunt and Uncle in 1939

At the end of the week we returned to my temporary Beckenham 'home' and it was almost at the end of the school holidays too. Unbeknown to me, arrangements had been made in London for my Uncle's school to be evacuated to Devonshire as soon as the anticipated War with Germany was declared and another change in my life occurred a few days later.

Late in the evening of Saturday, 2nd of September, my father arrived at my Aunt and Uncle's house. After closing the shop he had driven to Beckenham to collect my bits of luggage and my scooter, and take me to another 'home'. My Uncle's south London school was being evacuated almost immediately. Along with his pupils, my Aunt and Uncle also became evacuees. They had to pack up their essential belongings and travel with all the children to Devonshire for the duration of the War. Their own home was abandoned for six years and they lived in rented furnished accommodation until after the end of the War.

There were many civilian adults who were forced to leave their homes because of their jobs and spend the War in strange surroundings with new responsibilities. My Aunt, who had not worked outside her home since her marriage, was now occupied with the welfare of the evacuated children in Paignton and acting as a kind of untrained social worker. My relatives' comfortable detached house was damaged by the bombing during the Blitz, but when they made a brief visit to London to survey the War damage to their property they had no time to come and visit us. They had to get back to their charges in Paignton. It was dangerous in London at the time, their home was not fit to sleep in and they quickly returned to the safety of Devonshire.

I had to say a sudden, unexplained, but fond farewell to my relations. I didn't realise that I would not see them again for over six years. My father had been forced to find a new 'home' for me, and that evening I was on my way to yet another household.

Chapter SEVEN

FIRST MONTHS OF THE WAR

On the evening before War was declared, we set off on what seemed to me to be a long drive across London from Beckenham in Kent (now part of Greater London) to Mill Hill in North London. We arrived in the dark at the home of some elderly, distant relatives, although I only addressed them by their surname. I called them Auntie and Uncle Connell and never used their first names. My Uncle's name was Alfred, but I never knew what Auntie Connell's first name was. Even my father used to address them as 'Auntie and Uncle Connell'. They were a generation older than he was and they addressed each other as 'Mater' and 'Pater', not using a Christian name even when speaking to each other. It was a somewhat Dickensian household, exceedingly formal and restrained. They had two middle-aged sons; the elder one had emigrated to Australia and they never saw him again, although my Uncle was excited when he told us each Christmas that he had had a long distance 'phone call from 'Billy down under'. I met the younger son once when I was very tiny. My Uncle Connell drove my parents and me to the south coast to visit him, and I sat in the 'dickey' seat at the back of the car. The journey took so long, and I (hopefully) imagined that the sea was beyond the crest of every hill as I gazed ahead from my open seat. I was sure that the sky was the sea – another very early memory – and that our journey was nearly over! At last we reached a deserted seafront and drove along the road with a pebbly beach to our left until we reached a brand new petrol station on our right. Here I met this sort-of 'uncle' in the forecourt of his as-yet unopened business, no doubt anticipating the new wave of car owners driving to a developing seaside resort. I think it was Littlehampton. I wonder what the War did for his enterprise.

This Aunt and Uncle lived in a large detached house with a live-in maid named Olwen, and we had often visited them when my mother was well. Although I don't remember it, I have been told that I had lived with them for a while when I was very little - perhaps this was when I paid the visit to the seaside sitting in the little seat at the back of my Uncle's old-fashioned car? My Uncle Connell ran his own business as an industrial chemist and had commercial links in Germany prior to the War. He imported chemicals for the film industry, including the large Kodak factory near Harrow and other well-known companies. His trade with Germany came to an abrupt end with the outbreak of War. My parents had a holiday in Germany cruising down the Rhine with this Aunt and Uncle before I was born. Maybe it was combined with a business trip for my Uncle? (He was largely self-educated, had not had much formal education, or been to University, and was what used to be called a 'self-made man'; my Aunt and Uncle seemed to me to be quite 'grand'.) They had other old friends staying in the house on the night we arrived, who also referred to their hosts as 'Mater' and 'Pater' or 'Mr.' and 'Mrs. Connell'. These guests occupied all the spare bedrooms, so a camp bed was made up for me on the floor of my Uncle's dressing room.

The following morning was September 3rd, and after our Sunday breakfast the group of adults sat around in the morning room with solemn faces, anticipating the grave announcement shortly to be broadcast on the wireless. I can still recall the sense of doom and anxiety that was apparent on every face - my father, my Auntie and Uncle Connell, their neighbours, the elderly friends whom I called 'Auntie' Mabel and 'Uncle' Walter and 'Auntie' Alice. They had all lived through the First World War. Uncle Walter had been in the trenches and had been gassed; he had a bad chest and breathing difficulties, a quiet voice, and seemed weak physically. Auntie Alice had lost her sweetheart, still wore her engagement ring, but had never married. They were all too aware of what the nation was about to go through again. The atmosphere was strained - and smoky, as it always was at my Uncle Connell's. He was a habitual pipe smoker and the other men present smoked cigarettes.

Everyone, including Olwen, was present in the room that Sunday morning, listening intently to the wireless as the

Prime Minister made the announcement that 'this country is now at War with Germany'. I hovered somewhere around a large black lacquered screen that was usually placed across a draughty corner of the room, and I can still visualise all the adults who were seated in the easy chairs and around the table. It was frightening to hear the first air raid siren blasting out its warning of an imminent air raid - or so we all thought - shortly after the end of the broadcast. It turned out to be a false alarm, but everyone was very apprehensive, as almost immediate invasion was anticipated, and my Uncle hustled us all to the staircase that was built against the main inner wall of the house. This was considered to be a safe place in the event of a bomb falling nearby.

As we sat on the stairs, a person on each stair, one above another and close to the wall, Auntie Connell produced a box of Rowntree's Black Magic chocolates and handed them round, to distract us all, no doubt, from the fear of imminent annihilation! I can still remember the one I chose – the triangular shaped cream one - and always associate these chocolates with the outbreak of World War II. Eventually the haunting sound of the long, single tone of the 'All Clear' was heard; nothing terrible had occurred. Both the 'Alert' and the 'All Clear' were new sounds and rather weird and unnerving, but we would become accustomed to these sounds a few months later. We all descended from our various perches on individual stairs, and lunch was prepared and eaten in a rather subdued manner.

Life more or less resumed its usual pattern, but was never the same for anyone after that frightening announcement on the wireless. There was a sombre atmosphere surrounding the entire household. The neighbours went home and the visitors left after our Sunday lunch. At bedtime I slept in a proper bedroom of my own, next to Olwen's room. It had very dark, old-fashioned furniture, a large bed with an iron and brass bed-head end, plus a deep, fluffy feather mattress to snuggle into.

Olwen's little sitting room next to the kitchen was strengthened and made into an air raid shelter room shortly after this eventful day. Sandbags were stacked up, sticky tape stuck in a diamond pattern over the window and emergency supplies of staple foods were placed in the room. We all anticipated invasion, imminent air raids and gas attacks. Everyone had been issued with gas masks - horrible, smelly, rubber contraptions that we thankfully never had to use – and these were placed on a side table ready for immediate use. Food ration cards had been printed and distributed, and although rationing didn't come into force until the following year, I can recall seeing these official-looking books sitting on top of the sideboard in the dining room.

I lived at Mill Hill with my elderly Aunt and Uncle for some months. My Aunt wore old-fashioned, dull-coloured clothes with long skirts, and I thought she looked very ancient. My Uncle was a somewhat formidable-looking elderly gentleman, rather gruff and abrupt in speech, with a large moustache; he always seemed to have a pipe in his hand or his mouth. I became very fond of Olwen, a much younger woman than my Aunt. I preferred to be with Olwen in the kitchen, 'helping' her after she had washed up the dishes by sharpening the knives in an old drum-shaped sharpener. I inserted the clean knives into the individual slots of this piece of kitchen equipment (that one only sees nowadays in museums or National Trust House displays of 'downstairs life'). I turned the handle round and round to sharpen the non-stainless-steel blades. I followed Olwen around wherever she went, 'helping' her in whatever household task she was doing, and she was most patient and kind as I tagged along. She was very jolly and had a lovely dialect from her home county of Herefordshire.

I looked at and read as best I could some of my Aunt's very old Victorian books. She had kept these from her own childhood in the nineteenth century. The heavy books were placed on the table in front of me in the mornings; they were very large, printed with two columns to each page and looked rather like an old Family Bible. They contained a number of improving stories for young ladies, articles about good manners, etiquette and behaviour. The print was very small; many of the words were very long; a few pages had black-and-white illustrations. I have strong recollections of sitting on my own at the table in the morning room, quietly looking at, trying to read, and carefully turning, the pages of these rather boring, serious old books. I am sure they would have appeared uninteresting to any child of my generation, although no doubt they were considered admirable for Victorian young ladies' upbringing. Time passed slowly. I really preferred to be with Olwen in the kitchen, watching her preparing vegetables and scrubbing the soot and dirt off the celery as she chatted to me. It was much more interesting and companionable than old-fashioned books. I missed the interesting storybooks from my local Library.

I first heard the old adage "eat a peck of dirt before you die" in Olwen's soft country dialect. As we washed the vegetables at the sink we pondered together as to whether this meant a 'scrap' of dirt, or a 'peck' as in the old imperial measurement of weight, 'four pecks, one bushel'. The latter would have meant the consumption of a huge amount of dirt in a lifetime. Olwen was of the opinion that 'a little bit of dirt didn't do anyone any harm'! (Dirt in those days did not include chemical fertilisers, fungicides or insecticides; just soil, with maybe the addition of the household soot brushed down from the fire-back and the ashes from the grate.)

The kitchen in this house was tiny by any modern standard, with few fixtures or fittings and with little equipment. There was a dingy, ill-lit, walk-in larder and a small table by the side of a dark-green-painted dresser, which had shelves for china and some cupboard space beneath. A large solid fuel boiler provided all the hot water and a very minimal form of central heating in some of the rooms. The sink, the old gas stove and the cumbersome knife-sharpener seemed all-important and, together with the boiler, dominated the kitchen. Spacious, well-fitted kitchens were not thought important when this large house was built!

Whenever I opened the kitchen door I saw a strange looking, rusty old bicycle propped up against the outside wall. I didn't realise it at the time, but when I was older I recognised that it was a later model of a penny-farthing bicycle, presumably at one time ridden by my Uncle Connell. I would love to have seen him poised atop this weird vehicle, pedalling (or wobbling) down the road!

The dining room never seemed to have any sun shining through its windows, and consequently was rather gloomy. It was furnished with very large, solid oak, old-fashioned furniture. The sideboard had three enormous drawers in the middle and gleamed with its regular, energetic application of Olwen's 'elbow grease'. I used to help to lay the table for meals, getting the beautiful starched damask tablecloth and napkins, with their silver napkin rings, from one of the heavy drawers, and the old-fashioned, well-polished cutlery from another. A full-size bagatelle cabinet on four metal legs was tucked in the corner next to the sideboard. I spent many absorbing but solitary hours pulling the lever and releasing the heavy silvery metal balls one by one, watching them slip into their respectively numbered compartments, propped up by projecting pins, and then counting my score. There was nobody to compete with and it was a case of beating my own total. On the whole the days dragged by and life was very boring.

As a result of the War my Uncle's business was much reduced, and the following year the dining room was converted into my Uncle's office, but while I was living there we had all our meals at the large heavy oak dining table. On Mondays we always had what my Aunt called 'hash' for our mid-day dinner, which was the remains of the Sunday joint minced up and cooked with vegetables - the bottom part of a shepherd's pie! Olwen quite often placed a rabbit-shaped chocolate blancmange on the dining table for our dessert. It must have been made in the rabbit-shaped mould for my amusement, as I can't imagine either my elderly Aunt, or particularly my somewhat daunting Uncle, desiring chocolate blancmange in the shape of a rabbit for their pudding. I was always offered the first 'cut' of the rabbit and had to decide whether I would prefer the head or the tail, or even his plump middle, which was the biggest portion!

My parents and I once spent Christmas Day with these relations when I was four or five years old. Except that my mother was not among the group, the first Christmas of the War presented a similar picture. The same group of friends who were present at the previous Christmas house party, and who sat around the table when the War was declared, spent the holiday at Mill Hill. There was the same, smoky, slightly alcoholic atmosphere, although nobody drank to excess. (I always associated the smell of sherry, blended with an aroma of tobacco, with my Uncle Connell. The aroma seemed to mingle with his droopy moustache when I kissed him 'hello' or 'good-bye'.) As on that pre-War occasion, I was still the only child present in 1939, and I didn't really know what to do with myself. I can remember sitting on the floor in the dimly-lit room with very little to do but 'be seen and not heard', just looking at the logs crackling and occasionally spitting glowing fragments on to the carpet and making me jump. They burned brightly in the fireplace, scattering grey ash over the hearth, while the grown-ups chatted and smoked their cigarettes. I couldn't help casting my eye fearfully up to the top of the picture rail, above which was a pair of antlers, adorned with a holly branch. When I was little these antlers had seemed to me to be the whole head - perhaps it was the whole head - of a deer, that was peering down at me. I had been more than a little scared, but did not express my fear to this wholly adult party.

I don't remember any exchange of presents among the adults at Mill Hill, and indeed can't remember any presents I may have received myself on this occasion. It was the custom to have thinly-cut, cold roast beef sandwiches around the fire at midday on Christmas Day, at what seemed to me to be teatime. It may only have been lunchtime but the day dragged by so slowly that I was sure it was much later in the day. Christmas dinner was served in the evening. As the time for the meal drew near Auntie Connell disappeared into the kitchen with Olwen, who had been busy there all day. There was no room for me to join her on that special Day and get in the way, but delicious smells filled the house for several hours before we ate our Christmas dinner.

It was a very festive occasion, with the table beautifully laid with cutlery, napkins and cut glass wine glasses for all the adults. The table was decorated with a Christmas cracker for everyone. My Aunt carried in the turkey and Olwen followed with the vegetables and all the accompaniments were served in fine silver dishes. My Uncle carved the bird with much ceremony and skill. We pulled the expensive crackers, admired the little presents we found inside, the mottoes and jokes were read out and we put on our paper hats before we began to eat our meal. My rather intimidating Uncle, although a little brusque in his manner, was kindly and had a very dry sense of humour. He poured the white wine for the company, and as he, apparently casually, replaced the wine bottle on the very edge of the table, all the guests - including me, (this little drama was possibly done to amuse me) - gasped, as it nearly, but not quite, toppled over. He looked up, gazed calmly at us all and asked in a gruff voice "What's all this fuss about?" There was the bottle poised carefully just over the edge of the table, with its base ever so slightly unsupported. With a twinkle in his eye, he remarked, "I don't know what you're all getting so excited about". I was sure the bottle would fall over the edge of the table, as it was very precariously positioned. (This little performance was subsequently repeated every Christmastime during the War when, without fail, my father and I spent Boxing Day with my Auntie and Uncle Connell. There was no public transport on Christmas Day, so during the War our visit was made on the following day.)

After Olwen had cleared away our dinner plates, my Aunt carried in the Christmas pudding. Brandy had been poured over it and set alight, and the pudding was brought ceremoniously into the room surrounded by delicate flames. Exciting stuff for me! Even more exciting were the silver threepenny pieces and various other little silver trinkets that had been hidden in the pudding. As I ate my portion I was full of hope that I would be lucky enough to get one of these silver prizes - my wish was usually fulfilled. All the other guests at the table played up to the game of finding the little treasures in their portion of pudding, and our excitement was heightened when a little discovery was made as a spoon cut through a portion of pudding, alighted on something brittle, and a coin or a trinket was found. Such metal objects would be considered a health hazard nowadays, but gave much delight in days gone by.

Another custom of a visit to Mill Hill at Christmas was for the men to play billiards in the drawing room. Shortage of fuel prevented the drawing room from having a fire lit in the grate during the War and only the billiard players now used this room in the winter. A very small – not very efficient - portable electric fire was switched on. Maybe the men's absorption in their game of billiards (and the occasional glass of port or sherry) was considered to be enough to keep them warm! The ladies used to remain in the third reception room of the house - the morning room - where we had gathered when the War was declared. It was quite a large room, with not particularly attractive furniture, and the antlers were still above the picture rail, so I usually followed the men into the drawing room, perhaps wishing to be with my father to watch him play, or perhaps to get away from the antlers. I viewed the game silently, not daring to talk in the quiet but often intense atmosphere, as the men contemplated and played their strokes and then casually slid the peg along the scoreboard with their billiard cue to indicate each new total. When I got bored with the billiards, or had just grown cold, I quietly slid off to the warm kitchen to be with Olwen, or joined her in her little sitting room to chat.

The drawing room was still used on special occasions in the summertime. We sometimes had afternoon tea there when we visited my Aunt and Uncle. I can recall the brightness and attractiveness of this room, with the sun shining through the large bay windows, its wide-opened French-windows with flowery chintz curtains and furnishings. My Aunt had a china cabinet in this room and while the grown-ups were talking over their teacups I enjoyed inspecting all the interesting little objects displayed behind the glass. There were a number of miniature porcelain figures, tiny coffee cups and saucers and other knick-knacks that caught my attention, as well as the prettily decorated porcelain tea service. I then quietly slipped out of the room again to find Olwen making cakes in the kitchen.

She baked delicious little dark brown chocolate cakes from time to time and they were served still warm from the oven at teatime. I had never tasted homemade chocolate cakes before. In the coming years my father and I made occasional visits to these relations on Wednesday afternoons (his early closing day) or during my school holidays, and the gorgeous smell of freshly baked chocolate cakes sometimes wafted through from the little kitchen as we entered the house. The smell of chocolate cake still brings back memories of that period. Olwen sometimes bought what was called a mocha cake from the baker's shop. This coffee-flavoured iced cake had a sprinkling of chopped nuts round the edge; it was a real treat, and I am surprised that one could still buy such cakes in wartime. I had never eaten coffee cake before and had never even tasted real coffee at this time. The only coffee we drank when I was a child was the bottled 'Camp' variety, made from chicory root and sugar. This was a poor substitute for the real thing. Not many people drank fresh ground coffee in those days, and jars of freeze-dried instant coffee did not appear in the shops for some years.

Olwen always changed out of her 'working' clothes after the midday meal and I often sat on the bathroom stool while she washed. I think I must have clung to her like a leech! I still associate the smell of Pear's soap with my Auntie Connell's bathroom and Olwen's ablutions. When she had finished her morning's domestic duties and changed into her 'afternoon' dress we often walked to the shops together in Mill Hill Broadway. It was too far for us to carry all the shopping back home and most of our purchases were delivered.

I was once allowed to go to the pictures with Olwen on her 'evening off' to see 'Alexander's Ragtime Band'. As an eight-year-old it was a very special treat to be allowed to go to the evening film show at the local 'picture house', but I didn't really understand the film and thought the music was very loud, even though I loved it. I mostly enjoyed being allowed out late and walking home in the dark with my friend Olwen at the end of the evening.

Although she was 'in service' she had a pleasant, not over-stressed job, a nice home to live in, a comfortable bedroom and sitting room, but little independence and a rather solitary existence. Any thoughts of marriage or having children would have produced a dilemma - indeed this predicament occurred soon after the end of the War. (I think the gardener was involved and a baby boy was born.) The lovely drawing room became the living room for Olwen and her new baby. There was nowhere else for her to live for a while, as accommodation was hard to get after the War. My Aunt had died and my Uncle was very elderly. It was a long time before alternative care was found for him, and more appropriate accommodation for Olwen. I never discovered whether she married baby George's father. Olwen's home had been with my Aunt and Uncle since she left school and went 'into service'. Her offspring was the first small baby I had ever seen. When my father and I visited my Uncle I watched Olwen nursing little George with some curiosity and more than a little embarrassment as I wondered how she could have produced this infant, and what she was doing with him nuzzling at her breast. This was the only sight or experience of new babies I had in my childhood.

The enormous garden was my real delight. As well as the very large back garden, there were spacious grounds to the side and front of the house. There was a massive ancient oak tree in the middle of the front garden, casting a constant heavy shade, so the approach to the house was rather oppressive in those days. Ivy grew up the tree trunk and spread over the ground, which was smothered with a thick layer of dead leaves throughout the year. The front garden always seemed damp and gloomy. To the side of the house was a large, timber-framed greenhouse, but it seemed to be neglected and surprisingly little was grown in it while I was living there.

I preferred to wander round the various parts of the huge back garden, which had been laid out in different sections. There was a large lawn on either side of a central path. The lawn to the right had two mature weeping willow trees spreading their drooping branches over the regularly mown grass. I loved running through the long trailing branches of these seemingly mysterious trees. The lawn to the left of the path was the only dull section of the garden, with a nondescript evergreen tree planted in the middle of a small circular bed. I hardly ever walked on this lawn, which was heavily shaded by neighbouring trees, and consequently was very mossy and damp. Equally spaced rustic arches covered with climbing roses lined the garden path between the two lawns, which led me on to a beautiful garden full of different varieties of scented roses. Little paths edged with dwarf, scented box hedging surrounded the flowerbeds, which made a pleasing geometric pattern for me to run around. Memories of playing around these paths are always recalled whenever I smell old-fashioned roses or the subtle scent of box.

Leading on from the rose garden the path continued beside a deep flowerbed, which was filled with many brilliantly coloured dahlias of every shade, size and variety in the late summer and early autumn of 1939. A row of espalier peach trees was trained along a rustic trellis at the back of this large bed that produced a good crop of small, sweet peaches every season. In later years, if we were lucky enough to be visiting my Aunt and Uncle when the peaches were ripe, we came home with a big bag of the luscious fruit. These were much appreciated during the War when any kind of fruit was a treat and fresh peaches were a luxury never seen in the greengrocers' shops.

The path then wound its way down to a large goldfish pond with beautiful pink and white water lilies flowering in between the round lily pads that made a pattern on the surface of the water. During those September days I watched the iridescent dragonflies hovering and darting over and around the pond, their brilliant green or blue bodies glinting for an instant before they flew off to the irises and reeds at the edge. A little rustic bridge went across the narrower end of the pool leading to a less cultivated part of the garden, and beyond all this was the vegetable garden that I never entered. That was the gardener's domain. A little ornamental stream gently trickled down between rocks beside another path and into the pond. This path enabled me to make my journey back to the house by a different route. A deep pink flowering shrub grew against the back wall of the house. Olwen once told me it was a japonica. I couldn't get my tongue round this word when I was little and had called it a 'popinjay'. Olwen showed me the japonica (chaenomeles) in the autumn of 1939 with its branches laden with a large crop of unusual greenish fruits, which I still insisted on calling 'popinjays'.

I could almost get lost in this lengthy walk round the entire garden and certainly could not be seen by anyone from the house. It was my own little world. A lot of work was required to keep such a large garden so beautiful and productive, but I never saw my Uncle doing any gardening. He shared a gardener with his next-door neighbour, Mr. Elliott, who was a friend as well as a neighbour, and they often played billiards together. I rarely saw the gardener, and there must have been some reason unknown to me, some disability perhaps, as I don't think it was old age, which prevented him from being called up into the Forces. I often wondered where he lived, and assumed that he slept in the old garden shed beyond the rustic bridge!

I became familiar with so many different, often beautiful and fruitful gardens in my youth that must have had a strong influence on me in later years. I grew up to have a great interest in plants and gardens and am very fond of my own garden. It has given me so much pleasure over many years, although I am not quite so fond of the work it requires nowadays.

The house in which I lived during those first months of the War is still standing, but at least two detached houses have now been built in the grounds. The remaining garden must be so much smaller than in my childhood days; the pond and the willow trees will have gone; no doubt what remains is quite different, and, I am sure, is less interesting. The site is barely recognisable with the short access road and the additional large houses in what had been a beautiful garden.

The first few months of the War passed by quietly without incident in England. It was exceptionally quiet for me while I was living with my Auntie Connell, as I didn't see another child for the entire time I was there. Like most other school-age children still living in the London suburbs in the autumn of 1939, I received no education at all during the early months of the War. Most inner London pupils had been evacuated and most of the remaining schools were closed for some time during the early 'phoney' War period. Air raid shelters were already dug in some school playing fields, but these and other safety precautions took some time to complete. Lengthy ditches had to be dug out to house the pre-cast concrete tunnels that would provide protection (apart from any direct hit by a bomb), primitive sanitation and rough seating for entire school populations.

My mother did not appear to be recovering. I didn't talk about her, receive any messages from her after my father's Sunday visits, or overhear any conversation about her. I am sure it was considered best for me to be encouraged to forget her as quickly as possible; that after her last illness she was not expected to recover. I don't think my father believed that we would ever live together again as a family. This was largely true. I only thought of her occasionally in my day-to-day life, although in my prayers in bed at night I used to ask God to make my mother better, but we never lived together as a family after the summer of 1939.

When I saw her again twenty years later she seemed a stranger to me. She had begun to respond to the new anti-psychotic drugs that were introduced in the 1950s, and one Sunday I asked my father if I could accompany him on one of his visits to Shenley Hospital. The Staff agreed that it would be satisfactory for us to meet, and I went to the Hospital with my father and my younger son, who was still a baby. My father left me in the Hospital gardens while he went to her Villa and shortly returned accompanied by an elderly, white-haired lady. My parents walked across the grass together, and my mother and I greeted each other, but it all seems rather unreal to me now. I could accept her intellectually as my mother, but we did not recognise each other. We were complete strangers. It was a fairly tense meeting and I am sure we were all a bit nervous, but we talked together in a friendly way on a seat under an old oak tree. My mother fondled my son gently, but she didn't believe that he was her grandson. Neither could she accept that I was her daughter. Her courses of ECT seemed to have wiped from her memory any recollection of her past life that included me, and she never appreciated that she had a son-in-law, or two young grandsons, although she was interested in their activities and progress as they grew up.

From then on I accompanied my father on his routine, three-weekly visit. I saw that my mother was living in a pleasant environment and not in one of the old institutional workhouse-like asylums. From the early 1960s the whole family saw her frequently until her death in 1992. We grew fond of her. My sons called her 'Grandma', I called her 'Mumma' (my childhood name for her), she called me 'Sheila', but she never acknowledged our relationship. She once said to the Sister in charge of her Ward (or Villa) that she 'had had two daughters, "they" took both of them away'. In once sense this was true. She said she didn't know who I was, insisted that I was not her daughter, but told the Staff that I was her "best friend". Sister Brown encouraged her to accept our relationship, but I think this made her more adamant in asserting that I was not her daughter. I talked to her about my Aunt, who was her sister, my Uncle, who was her brother-in-law and other relatives. I chatted about the few incidents remembered from my childhood when she was at home, but to no avail. She was unable to make the connection between the child she had been suddenly separated from, and me as a married woman. She appeared content with her restricted life, appreciated our visits, always had a good appetite, even managing to eat roast meat without any difficulty without any teeth, although I never found out why all her teeth had been removed, or why she had never been fitted with dentures.

After my father died in 1982 my husband and I began taking in 'afternoon tea' to my mother when we visited her, and the Staff allowed us to use a small side room. I laid a small table with an embroidered tablecloth, and brought a flask of hot water to make tea, which I poured into my parents' old 'best' china teacups, which I had brought with me. We ate dainty sandwiches, homemade cake, chocolate éclairs, or strawberries and cream, and my mother declared that 'it's like a "young Christmas" every time you come to see me'! It was a very simple pleasure, but was obviously such a treat for her to drink a freshly made cup of tea from nice china, and to eat non-institutional food. I often think of the depravations she endured for so much of her lifetime, and the indignities she may have suffered.

Middlesex County Council developed Shenley Hospital in 1934 on the site of a large eighteenth century Manor House and Country Estate in Hertfordshire. A banker who was said to suffer "severe delusions of grandeur" owned the original imposing House. He added a number of ornate features and built a beautiful impressive cupola. The House was turned into a recuperation centre for shell-shocked soldiers during the First World War, and further extensions were made before the more modern Mental Hospital was designed and built by John Laing, the large building construction company, before the Second World War.

The Manor House, called 'Porter's Mansion', was begun in the 16th century and is a Grade 2 listed building, situated on the highest point in southern Hertfordshire. Patients knew it as 'The Mansion' but I never knew to what purpose it was put when it was part of Shenley Hospital. Many of the large old specimen trees growing on the original Estate were retained in the beautifully landscaped grounds surrounding the Wards or 'Villas', as they were called. Each Villa could accommodate between 20 and 45 men or women patients. Although in a lovely rural area, Shenley Hospital was situated a long way away from the North London suburbs it was designed to serve. Relatives had a difficult journey by public transport from Harrow or Wembley in order to visit a patient. Was it anticipated that not many family members would in fact visit, and that many long-term patients would actually be abandoned and forgotten? Shenley Hospital housed up to 2000 patients in these Villas, each with its own open garden area where patients could sit or take a walk in the spacious grounds, if the Staff felt they were able.

The Wards had locked doors for many years in case very disturbed patients attempted to get out. The Sister had the key, and when I began to visit my mother in the l960s the unobtrusive entrance door to her Ward was occasionally locked, and when my father and I arrived we had to ring the bell in order to be admitted. The development of anti-psychotic drugs gradually made patients more controllable and less disturbed, and subsequently the system became more relaxed. With modern knowledge of the bad effects of institutionalisation of psychiatric patients (and possibly political money-saving policy) the Hospital was slowly run down in the l990s. Older, long-term patients like my mother died and others were returned to the care and responsibility of their families, hopefully with adequate support and supervision. The rest were dispersed into smaller, supervised homes or discharged into community care (?).

My mother did at least spend the last tragic fifty-three years of her life in one of the most modern, well-built and hopefully more enlightened Hospitals of the last century. Perhaps she was better cared for than many other mentally ill people in that period. She was possibly safer and more contented than some who nowadays may receive inadequate care, but I believe that she endured much deprivation, rather Spartan conditions in the earlier years, some harshness and little homeliness for many of the years she lived there. Nursing mentally ill patients was an exceedingly difficult occupation or calling before the advent of the modern drug therapies. It is still hazardous and requires special talents.

Shenley Hospital was finally closed in 1999 and the entire site has been developed for privately owned residential housing, while retaining some of the original landscaping and many of the beautiful trees. There is now a small group of shops and a local purpose-built Surgery to care for the medical needs of the new residents of what is now called Porters Park. A South African award-winning interior designer bought the Mansion in 1998 but it changed ownership again soon afterwards.

All that remains of the old Hospital are the Mansion, the Chapel, the Clock Tower, the Orchard and the Walled Garden. The Clock Tower disguised the water tower in former years and is still a very visible landmark dominating the skyline for miles around. The Chapel is now available to the residents in the new community for various functions, but sadly is not used as the local community church. The old apple trees in the Orchard still produce fruit from almost one hundred different varieties of apples.

The huge Walled Garden dates back to the 16th century, and, with the protection given by the high walls, thirty-five gardeners were employed in the early years of Shenley Hospital to help to make the Hospital self-sufficient. Gardening has always appeared to be a very useful form of therapy and with the assistance of many of the male patients the Walled Garden supplied the Hospital with all its fruit and vegetables during the War. It was gradually run down and eventually grew into disuse long before the Hospital closed. The Walled Garden has now been wonderfully restored and transformed, with a series of terraces with wide grassy paths and borders of shrubs and flowers. A grassy amphitheatre has been formed in the lower, eastern side of the old garden, where open-air concerts and events take place in the summer. It is managed by the Shenley Park Trust and is open to the public. One can now look out on the rural Hertfordshire countryside beyond the old walls whilst enjoying the beauty of the Garden.

Another part of the old Hospital complex has been developed as a rural Park with car parking and toilet facilities, walks and a tearoom; The Pavilion was opened in the summer of 2001. When visiting the new Estate I can just make out where my mother's last residential Villa was situated. The whole landscape has changed, with the exception of most of the large old trees, which enhance the area. With all this new development it is difficult to imagine the Shenley Hospital I knew for so many years. My late parents would find it unbelievable!

It was the end of an era when the Hospital finally closed its doors to the mentally ill, and, although medication for psychiatric illness is now much improved from when my mother was first affected, I wonder whether psychiatric care is now better. Certainly, if my mother had been born fifty years later, it is unlikely that she would have had to spend most of her adult life in a mental institution. I am not convinced that her care would have been better, or that the strain, uncertainty and perhaps fear of looking after her at home, might not have resulted in both my parents suffering from some nervous affliction. Could my father have coped? Long-term institutional care means no quality of life for the patient. Improved diagnosis, better understanding of the various kinds of mental illness, and improved medication appear to be the best ways forward, but there seem to be no answers to some of life's problems.

There used to be so much shame and blame attached to both the patients and the relatives of those with mental illness or mental disability and this has still not been totally removed from society. Even in the nineteen-fifties, mental handicap was not openly spoken about, as Sir Brian Rix knew from the experience he had with his Down's syndrome daughter,

Shelley. His father never spoke to his son about his granddaughter after her birth, and never consented to see her. Shelley herself has lived her life in an institution. This terrible stigma was attached to any illness or disability of the mind or the nerves or the brain. I am sure it was more extreme in the last century but it still exists today. I believe that it was to protect me from this perceived shame that my father and my relatives, rightly or wrongly, thought it best to encourage me to forget my mother.

Sometimes a sense of guilt or responsibility for the illness was placed on the relatives of the mentally ill. It was considered by some in those early days of the last century that brain damage, epilepsy and other neurological conditions were caused through the parents' bad habits or sinful behaviour. Had this sense of shame been unwittingly placed on either or both of my parents after the birth and early death of my sister Peggy? Did my mother have to live with this stigma on top of the sorrow of losing her first baby? I do hope not. I will never know the answers to these questions.

My father continued to live at our house in Kenton during the months I spent with my Aunt and Uncle. He was still able to use his car in the early days of the War and he saw me most Sundays after he had been to see my mother. Her condition wasn't mentioned in my hearing and I didn't like to ask about her, but I used to ask him how Betty, our Airedale dog, was. He told me he had to leave her outside in the garden all day while he was at work and that she was getting out of control with nobody to look after her or take her for walks. When I next enquired about Betty I was told that she had been given away to another family. I had a shrewd suspicion even as a child that she had been taken to the vet and been put down. I never asked any more questions about her.

When I returned to my own home, not only was my mother not there, Betty had gone and the garden was wrecked. Sadly, Roy and Olive who had lived next door had been evacuated to Australia and their parents had moved. My friend Johnny Boughton who had been to tea with me, and

David, with whom I had made mud pies, no longer lived along the road with his sister Irene. They had all been evacuated. Everything had changed.

Chapter Eight

HOME AGAIN

Time passed by and my mother did not appear to be recovering. I am sure my father was consumed with anxiety about her and concerned about how he was going to cope with bringing me up. The long hours of work required in the retail trade, and the all day opening of the shop on Saturday made it difficult for him to look after me. There was no help in those days; no adjustment of working hours for extenuating circumstances, or assistance from Social Services.

My father also had a number of financial worries. I have no idea how the cost of my mother's long-term (for the rest of her life) residence in a Mental Hospital was met before the National Health Service was introduced. He had a mortgage to pay on our Kenton house and another mortgage on our previous home at Osterley. He had rented this house to a spinster lady as an investment when we moved in 1935. This might have seemed a good business venture in 1935, to continue to pay the mortgage, get an income from the rent and assume that the value of the house would increase, but it was certainly not such a good idea in 1939 or 1940. Rents were controlled during the War and nobody was allowed to raise them for many years afterwards. During the coming years I remember my father saying, with some passion, that the Osterley house was 'a millstone round my neck'. From time to time he received letters from his elderly tenant, asking for payment for the repair of burst pipes, or a broken fence, blocked drains, or some other maintenance and he didn't know how to find the money to pay these bills. He was unable to rid himself of the burden of that house until well into the 1950s.

He had been forced to wind up "Percy's", his small menswear shop in Southall. He could not find a suitable replacement Manager after Mr. Wookey was called up, but he knew the clothing trade would suffer during the War, so he closed his shop and lost money. He retained his position as Manager of Meakers, but with fewer customers buying less clothing, income was comparably lower too, because shop assistants added to their wages by commission on sales. He had come upon hard times. Although I was only a child at the time I had an awareness of his worries over 'making ends meet' and his general anxiety. Everything seemed to have turned against him and from his rising status and comparative prosperity; he had now lost so much.

He had to find a way of providing some kind of settled home life for both of us. I can now appreciate that I might have found myself fostered in a long-term placement, or been put into a children's home, but he managed to find a way out. I soon learned that we were to have a 'housekeeper', but it was with great difficulty that my father managed to afford to pay her. I didn't know what a 'housekeeper' was and I certainly did not understand the intensity of his many problems at the time, but I soon began to sense his tension and worry after I returned to my old home.

He arrived at my Auntie Connell's house one weekend and told me that I was going home. My belongings were packed; I said my farewells to my Aunt and Uncle, and to dear Olwen who had so patiently allowed me to trail around after her as she did her housework. She was always so cheery and companionable and I was sorry to leave her. I returned to Kenton with my father and saw my own home again for the first time for many months. The housekeeper and her daughter were already in the house when I arrived home and another new phase began in my life.

I had no prior understanding of this new development, or any explanation as to what our future family life was to be. It was an experiment for all concerned. My first memory is of meeting the housekeeper and her daughter in our dining room and feeling very shy with these two strangers. Rose and I sat uncomfortably squashed together on the seat of one of the old leather, velvet-cushioned armchairs, while our respective parents talked to each other. Our own conversation was a bit

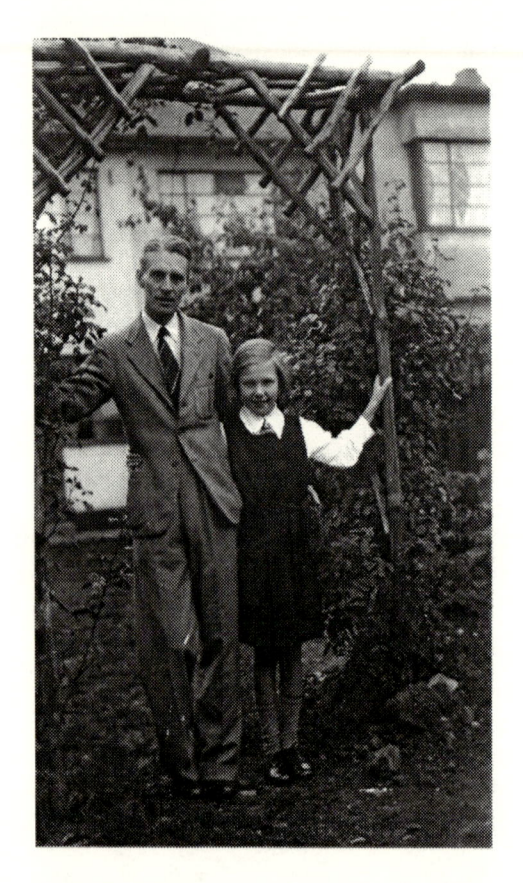

With my father in the garden in 1940.

strained, but I learned that Rose was in her second year at Senior School. I had completed my first year of Junior School in the summer. Later on I learned that she had not seen her father since she was a small child. He was not in the Forces, but lived in another continent. I don't believe she was in contact with him, or ever saw him again. I now realise that Rose and I were both minus a parent, and it seems strange that we never spoke to each other about our absent father or mother. It didn't appear to make a particular bond between us, which I am sure would occur nowadays.

'Auntie', as I was soon to call her mother, suggested that she went into the kitchen to make us all a cup of tea. I didn't like tea and had never drunk it until that day, but I could not pluck up the courage to say that I didn't want to have tea. I was given a cup of tea without sugar in it and drank it up, and from that time on I drank tea and soon grew to enjoy it. I have never had sugar in it, although in those days most people added sugar to their tea. Soon after food rationing came into force our housekeeper wished she had more sugar to use in cooking. My father, who was the only one in our new household to take sugar in his tea, agreed to sacrifice his spoonful of sugar, and we were surprised to find how much sugar had dissolved away unnoticed in cups of tea during a week! I think that the deprivation of sweetened tea was the least of his concerns.

We soon got to know each other and settled down together quite harmoniously. The housekeeper and Rose shared what had been my large back bedroom and for a while I slept in a makeshift bed on the floor in my father's (what had been my parents') bedroom. My mother's silver-backed mirror and hairbrush were still displayed on the dressing table, with a cut-glass powder-bowl to one side, and another bowl on the other side still contained her powder puff. I sometimes went into the bedroom in the daytime and sat on the stool in front of the dressing table. I lifted the lid, smelt the powder in the bowl and brushed the soft fluffy swansdown puff against my cheek. At either end of the dressing table were round silver photograph frames containing sepia pictures of two old ladies.

I often looked at these and wondered who these old ladies were, but nobody had ever talked to me about my grandparents and at that time I didn't know who or what grandmas were! I don't remember consciously missing my mother, but I believe I was a little bewildered and didn't understand what was happening and often spent some time alone in the bedroom.

In the bottom of the wardrobe I found my mother's fox fur stole. It was a fashionable, and in those days, an acceptable accessory for a lady to wear over her coat when going out. My mother used to drape the fox's fur around her neck and then clasp the tail on to a little metal clip attached to the fox's head. I often sat on the floor in front of the wardrobe, hidden by my parents' double bed, stroking the fur and patting the hard little head. Perhaps I recalled seeing my mother wearing her stylish little fox fur wrap, but she was gradually becoming a remote figure in my life...but I think I was missing something. I don't know what happened to all her clothes.

My father eventually obtained a single bed for me, which was put in what we always called 'the little room' over the hall; I now had my own bedroom once more, with a proper bed instead of the mattress on the floor of my father's room. His small fitted gentleman's wardrobe was brought into the room for my use. One didn't require much storage space in those days of limited clothing.

Some semblance of school life was resumed after Christmas. In the New Year our teachers began to arrange lessons for small groups of children in various homes in the immediate neighbourhood. We had all had a continual 'holiday' since the beginning of September. I began to have brief lessons with a few of my old classmates once or twice a week in a house not very far from my own home, but we didn't learn very much. We sat around in chairs in somebody's cold living room, with exercise books propped on our knees, trying to do our sums or some written work for an hour or two. I didn't recognise any of my old classmates. It all seemed like a game, too informal, too uncomfortable and so unimportant. Eventually school reopened, but no sooner had we settled in our classes and begun to catch up on reading, arithmetic (not maths in those days!) and other basic subjects, than the Battle of Britain began in the summer of l940 and air raids disturbed our days at school and our nights' rest too.

A large Kodak factory (supplied with some of its essential chemicals by my Uncle Connell's business) was only a couple of miles away in Wealdstone, producing, developing and printing film for the War effort. There were also a number of 'shadow' factories in the (not immediate) vicinity, which had been commercial premises and car showrooms. They were requisitioned by the Ministry of Aircraft Production to give additional facilities to the de Havilland Engine Company's large factory at Edgware, helping to increase their capacity to produce, repair and overhaul aircraft engines. Consequently we had many air raids and a number of bombs fell in the Harrow area.

An RAF Barrage Balloon Station was established in Stanmore about three miles to the North of our house and in a different direction from the factories. The Headquarters of Fighter Command was also situated in Stanmore, on part of the large Bentley Priory Estate, and the Operations Room had secretly been built underground just before the War started. A large area of the surrounding woodland and countryside remained open to the public throughout the War, but the civilian population had no idea of the vital work being carried out nearby beneath the ground. Sir Hugh Dowding directed the Battle of Britain from here during 1940 and 1941. These factors may also have contributed to some of the enemy activity in our area. Nobody knew where the anti-aircraft guns were situated, or who manned them, but we were very much aware of the 'ack-ack' of the gunfire during the air raids. Belmont Hill was about a mile away from our house, and Harrow Hill was only a couple of miles away; both seem probable sites for the gun emplacements. I often saw the barrage balloons in the sky to the north of our home during the daytime. Whether they were being tested at the RAF

Station, or whether they were intended to protect Fighter Command I do not know.

I don't think I took much notice of the progress of the War, although I can remember the grave attention that was paid to the news bulletins on the wireless each day. Children were not well informed about the War situation, and our understanding about politics, current affairs, disasters, or wars, was negligible compared with that of young people nowadays. Television makes all news much more accessible. Perhaps, when one was so closely involved, it may have been better for us to remain in some ignorance, but I now feel that I didn't receive enough background knowledge of the historical period I lived through.

I recall walking home from school one day with my friends. We were all singing La Marseillaise - in French - at the tops of our voices, much enjoying the stirring tune but not understanding the meaning of the words of the French National Anthem. We had learned this song at the time of the fall of France and were possibly told something of the seriousness of this event in the classroom, but I can only remember singing the song with gusto. We were not taught French at school and had merely learned the words by rote. I have very faint memories of hearing on the BBC Home Service News bulletin about the fall of Dunkirk and the small boats rescuing the soldiers, but I had no idea of what was actually happening.

It was shortly after the Dunkirk rescue that the Battle of Britain began. As soon as the siren sounded during the daylight raids, all the children were led with much urgency into the long air raid shelters that had been dug in our school field. We all carried our gas mask in a cardboard box slung over our shoulders, with a little tin of emergency 'rations' inside, only to be consumed in a serious crisis. We sat back-to-back on the rough wooden benches that had been fixed along the middle of the tunnel of the shelter, and spent hours playing noughts and crosses, 'hangman', or 'boxes' on little scraps of paper, using up every inch of space with our pencil and paper games. 'Boxes' took up the longest time, with the preliminary marking out of a rectangle of equally spaced dots, followed by each player joining up two dots, and eventually completing a square - or 'box' - which was marked with the appropriate initial. Often, if one was perceptive, it was possible to gain a good number of 'boxes', and the simple game did help to while away the long, boring, sometimes chilly, hours in the shelters. 'Cat's cradle' was another game we played with a length of wool or string. It was another way of passing the time, and later became one of the annual 'crazes' in the various games that suddenly became popular during the school year. We also sang 'counting' songs such as 'Ten Green Bottles', 'This Old Man, He Played One', which kept our spirits up and helped to pass the time.

If an air raid went on for a very long time, the teachers handed boiled sweets around, but little or no teaching was possible in the shelters. It was not light enough to read a book. The facilities were very basic and unpleasant if anyone wanted to go to the toilet, only a bucket and some disinfectant. I don't remember using it. I guess I just 'held it'. Normal lessons were very irregular and infrequent during these months.

In the anxious months before the start of the War, manufacturers and retailers of household fabrics must have made a fortune selling strong, black curtain material, and there must have been a frenzy of activity by anxious housewives throughout the country, making black linings for their curtains. Regulations came into force as soon as War was declared and everyone had to make sure that no light could be seen through their windows after dark. Not a chink of light was allowed to shine through any windows to indicate to German bombers that there was a built-up area, factory or dwelling-place down below. Curtains, shutters, old blankets or some other makeshift screening had to cover every window before a light was switched on. I remember our windows at home being covered with criss-crossed sticky tape to help to prevent them shattering if a bomb fell nearby, but I can't remember my mother making these curtains before the War.

I wonder whether the anxiety and apprehension in those pre-war months could have caused the severe recurrence of her mental condition?

However, we certainly had blackout curtains, which were drawn across our windows very carefully every evening at dusk, making sure that not a single gap allowed a glimpse of light to show through. Air Raid Wardens, recruited from men too old to be called-up, or those in reserved occupations, were on regular duty looking out for any chinks of light, glimmers glowing through, or even a blaze of light from un-drawn curtains. 'Put that light out' was a common phrase of those times. We didn't dare put a light on in a room before the curtains had been pulled across the windows. Factories and offices had to be equally vigilant. Any vehicle on the road (there were not many cars, as petrol was soon rationed and available only for essential use) travelled with masked headlights at night. All streetlights were extinguished for the duration of the War. Direction signs had also disappeared for fear of invasion, so any kind of travel by road in unfamiliar areas was a little hazardous. Pedestrians carried small hand torches to enable them to find their way along darkened streets. These were carefully directed down to the pavement and never raised up towards the sky.

We carried our gas masks wherever we went, to work, to school, to the shops, to the pictures and to Church, but as the War progressed the fear of gas attacks receded and we began to leave them at home. I hated the horrible black rubber mask, which clung to my face, smelt disgusting and made my voice sound strange when talking, but the only time we put them on was when we had occasional gas mask practices in the classroom at school.

My father was an Air Raid Warden, and took his turn of night duty on the rota for fire-watching, looking out for light showing from inadequately or un-drawn curtains, as well as dealing with any small fires from incendiary bombs. He had his tin hat, bucket and stirrup pump, but I never knew if his services had been required in the night when incendiary bombs were dropped, or even where his area of patrol was. These activities were not talked about the following morning and I had no idea of how often, or how much of the night, he had spent walking the streets in his ARP duties.

Many air raids occurred at night, with the ominous sound of the siren blaring out its warning tones of approaching enemy aircraft waking us all from sleep. At the start of the Blitz our household of four used to lie on the floor of our drawing room, close to the chimneybreast. That was considered to be the strongest and so the safest part of the house and the least likely to be demolished if there was a direct hit. We lay on mattresses that had been dragged downstairs and placed on the floor, and covered ourselves with our eiderdowns. Thankfully, we did not experience any bombing in the immediate vicinity, nor did we sustain any damage to our house, but we heard the German bombers coming over, and the 'ack-ack' fire from the anti-aircraft guns soon joined the throbbing noise of the approaching bombers as the gunners sought to bring them down. The sound of the firing seemed to be everywhere, but it grew more frightening when the sound of the bombers' engines was overhead; sometimes followed by the awful heart-stopping fear when the whine or whistling sound was heard as a bomb hurtled down, with the sudden ground-shaking thud of the ensuing explosion.

We thought we could judge the distance and direction of the bomb in rather the same way that we estimated the number of miles away the thunderclap is in a thunderstorm -by counting the seconds after the lightning flash - ...'I wonder where that one fell?' went through our minds. The bomber seemed to be more or less overhead but one could tell by the degree of ground shake, the volume of noise from the explosion, whether the bomb was a little distance away or much further off. The sound of the German bombers was also unnerving, with an unusual, heavy, irregular throb of the engines.

Sometimes there were long quiet periods during a raid when we tried to doze off for a while. If the 'All Clear' blasted out during the night there was then the possibility of a few hours' sleep before going to work or school next morning. However, the likelihood of sleep was reduced in our family, as I was a very heavy tooth grinder. I started another kind of ordeal for the family as soon as I had dozed off to sleep and kept everybody else awake with the grinding of my teeth as we lay on the floor in our drawing room. I sometimes woke myself up with the noise I made and can still sense the heavy weight that bore down on my jaws and teeth from the pressure I was creating. Snoring is an awful sound, but I think that teeth grinding may be even worse. I had this habit for many years of my childhood.

Part of the lawn in our back garden that had been lovingly sown and nurtured by my parents a few years previously was now dug up to make a proper air raid shelter, to give us a safe haven in the event of a bomb falling nearby or on the house. I can recall nothing of the removal of the turf, or the deep hole that my father dug into the clay soil of our lawn. Somehow or other he fixed the curved, corrugated iron panels of this semi-underground shelter into position, and heaped the soil over the semi-circular hump showing above the ground. We tried unsuccessfully to grow marrows in the soil piled up at the end of this air-raid shelter, but without much success. My father fitted rough wooden bunks inside and made a little door that we shut behind us when we had stepped down into the 'dungeon' at the start of an air raid. This small shelter, 4ft.6in.x 6ft. x 6ft. (the size of a very small greenhouse) was supposed to accommodate up to six people! I understand the cost of this prefabricated kit was £7, but that it was offered free to those householders who earned less than £250 a year. I was never informed of my father's income and don't know whether he qualified for a free kit. The shelter had been designed and approved by the Government, and named after the then Home Secretary and Minister of Home Security, John Anderson, later Lord Waverley. He became Chancellor of the Exchequer in 1943 and subsequently introduced PAYE.

As soon as we heard the whine of the siren waking us from our sleep we tumbled out of our beds, and grabbed something warm before trailing down the garden path to the shelter. We were squashed close together in the dark, and it was impossible to sleep. When the 'All Clear' sounded hours later, we crawled out of the tiny door, thankful to see our home still standing. We were shocked to see the sky was very bright with reflections from the incendiary bombs dropped on the Docks in London when we scrambled out into the fresh air in the early hours of one morning. The flare from the flames of various local fires in the nearby gardens was alarming too. Rose and I pranced around the garden in our nightdresses in the middle of the night, before dancing up the garden path to the kitchen door, excited by the strange atmosphere, but not understanding the danger and loss of life and home that many had suffered. We had been squeezed together in the dark, damp, semi-underground shelter for hours, and seemed to behave as if it was some kind of Guy Fawkes celebration. Maybe we were both over-reacting to the atmosphere of this extraordinary night when we were suddenly let loose into the unnatural brightness created by the incendiary bomb flames and the reflections against the night sky. We had no understanding of the damage to the London Docks that night. The remembrance of the dampness, the darkness, the chill and the dank air of that dugout shelter remain with me still. It was awful. Equally strong is the memory of the unnatural brightness of the night. Shortly after this we abandoned the shelter and remained in our own beds throughout the night raids.

Children had a rather curious pastime on the mornings after a bad air raid. As we walked to school we peered at the pavement, crept into people's driveways, looked in the gutters and along the grass verges, searching for bits of shrapnel from a bomb or shell case that had exploded in the night. I kept a large collection of these pieces of contorted metal in a drawer for many years as a rather odd souvenir. With hindsight it appears to have been a very bizarre kind of interest, but it was a fascinating hobby for young school children at the time and our shrapnel collections were much prized.

One would have thought that only factories, businesses, food shops, essential travel, emergency, medical and maintenance services would have continued during this period, but life seemed to proceed as usual. People took shelter as best they could in the night, slept when they were able, and kept life as normal as possible during the daytime. Children went off to school the following morning, spent long periods of the day in the shelters and accepted the current circumstances as ordinary everyday life.

As time went on we became almost immune to the dangers of the night raids that continued for some time after we had abandoned the Anderson shelter, which gradually filled with water and became quite uninhabitable. We continued to remain indoors in our own beds rather than use the alternative communal brick shelters that had been built in many streets. At times I crept out of bed during an air raid and stood on the lino looking out of my window at the night sky. I watched the searchlights making patterns, as their beams of bright light darted and criss-crossed in the dark sky, endeavouring to pinpoint an enemy plane.

During one of the major air attacks on London, we all got out of bed and stood in our nightclothes at the back bedroom window, gazing in awe mixed with horror at the huge red glow of the distant flames, and watched in disbelief as London burned. The conflagration was so great from the incendiaries and high explosives, and it was really horrifying to see the sky glowing ominously so far away in the City of London.

The Battle of Britain had started in early August 1940 and the attempt was made to destroy London and the morale of those living and working in the capital by continuous raids between September 7th and October 5th. It was one of these raids that produced the truly awesome and unforgettable sight we saw in the sky that night. Hitler could not destroy the spirit of the people in London, and the brave airmen who fought and won the Battle of Britain saved our country from invasion. The Blitz continued more unpredictably for many months after this intense period of bombardment, but Raids did not occur on every single day and night as the season passed into winter of 1940 - a very bitter one - then through to the spring of 1941.

The local bombing I experienced was in no way to be compared with the destruction in London and some other major cities. We did not have whole streets flattened or even bombs in every road, but there were quite a number of bombed-out homes in the locality that became semi-empty spaces, and there was much enemy activity in the air, with consequent defensive fire.

I had a recurrent bad dream during these months and at subsequent times during the War that I have been unable to forget. I never experienced any machine-guns firing from low-flying enemy aircraft, but I had probably seen pictures on the newsreel at the cinema, perhaps at the time of the evacuation of Dunkirk, when there was continual strafing, and the sight of the low-flying planes together with the sound of the machine-gun fire may have been impressed on my mind. In my nightmare I had come out of my house, shut the front door, only to hear the sound of very low-flying aeroplanes in the distance where the barrage balloons were often seen. As I looked up the road, I saw in my dream three large, dark aircraft zooming low, fast and very loud, just above the rooftops. I stood in the little recess on our open-fronted porch, where the milkman used to place our bottles of milk. I tried to conceal myself in this small space, kicking the bottles out of the way, but realising that I was unable to hide, and was still facing up the road with the planes flying towards me, their machine guns firing rapidly. As they flew by I woke up with a mixture of fear and relief. This brief nightmare recurred many times, but the fear seemed to linger for much longer. Perhaps in my sleep I was hearing the local anti-aircraft guns firing and this was turned into a bad dream. My bedroom was over the hall and above the porch and the corner where my bed was placed was in a similar position to the alcove in the porch beneath. This may have accounted for some of the extreme reality of this oft-repeated dream. I never told anyone about it and can recall no other dream that I had in my childhood after such a long period of time.

My father used to come into my room each morning and wake me up. For many years his greeting was a bright, "Wakey, wakey, show a leg there; the sun's scorching your eyes out". This was a morning 'greeting' remembered from his First World War service days, when the men were brusquely roused from slumber in their barracks. On bright mornings he sometimes sang a little song about the sun, "The sun has got his hat on, hip, hip, hip, hooray; the sun has got his hat on and is coming out today". It was a cheerful start to the day, but I often required a second call, and have always been more of an owl than a lark. I was not eager to get up in the mornings - especially in the cold, dark days in the winter when the sun was NOT shining!

Once I had plucked up my courage to drag myself from under the bedclothes and set foot on the cold linoleum of my bedroom floor, I rushed to the bathroom to get washed and dressed. The wide-open airing cupboard door was very welcome in the winter, allowing the warmth from the hot water tank to be added to the heat produced by the towel rail. I hurried down to the kitchen, where, hopefully, the boiler had remained alight throughout the night and had kept the room warm. After my father had raked it and topped it up with coke, it was usually burning away brightly. 'Auntie' pulled the damper out to encourage some little flames, and opened the little door at the front, so that we could see as well as feel the heat from the coke glowing behind the grid as we ate our breakfast.

We take our centrally heated homes so much for granted nowadays - although I often say a quiet 'thank you' for my warm home and do appreciate its comfort.

Chapter Nine

GOING TO CHURCH

I recall very little about daily life with our housekeeper and her daughter in the first year or so after 'Auntie' and Rose became part of our household, apart from the recollections of how we coped in the air raids. The sirens, bombing, gunfire, shelters and 'all clear' were in the forefront of all our minds at that time. However, I do remember going to Church and Sunday School. 'Auntie' and her daughter had attended a small non-conformist church on Sundays before she started working for my father, and they continued to go to the services after they came to live with us. I'm not sure what I amused myself with on Sunday mornings while Rose and her mother were at church, although I can quite clearly recall sitting at the dining table reading Max Miller's jokes page in my father's Sunday Dispatch newspaper while he was gardening or doing household jobs.

My memory of Sunday mornings when my mother was well and at home was of my parents having a 'lie in' and a cup of tea in bed whilst reading the paper. My father went down to the kitchen to make this morning tea, and when I heard him bringing it upstairs I slipped out of my own bedroom and climbed into my parents' bed amidst the rustle of the newspaper and the stirring of tea. I waited expectantly for the bar of Cadbury's Caramello filled-block chocolate that I knew my father would produce for me each week. This was *my* Sunday treat. I was never disappointed. Sometimes I had a bar of Aero chocolate and I was content with either of these chocolate bars while my parents drank their morning tea. But those days had gone.

After the worst of the Blitz was over, 'Auntie' suggested to my father that I accompanied her and her daughter on Sundays, so I began to join them in their walk to church each week. Their little church was not unlike my wooden primary school to look at, both rather surprising structures in a suburban area of contemporary housing, and both were, no doubt, ex-army huts put to peaceful uses after the First World War. We lived about a mile away from the church, which was situated on the edge of a large council estate and affectionately known to the congregation as 'The Hut'! After a brisk twenty minutes walk along streets of small, neat, modern houses we reached the little prefabricated building. We often arrived shortly after the service had begun and had to stand waiting in silence in the tiny vestibule for what seemed a very long time until the lengthy opening prayer was over. We always hurried along, trying to get to the service before 11a.m., but we might as well have taken our time over the dinner preparations at home, walked a little less hurriedly and arrived some minutes later. We could then have gone straight in and found our seats after the end of the long extempore opening prayer, because we were nearly always late - and this first prayer was always so *long*.

We always had a rush on Sunday mornings, eating breakfast hurriedly before washing the dishes, preparing the dinner and putting the little joint and potatoes in the oven before we left home. When fresh peas were in season during the summer, Rose and I were given the task of shelling them before our walk to church. We carried a tray, a colander and a brown paper bag of peas down the garden path and sat in the sun in our best 'Sunday' dresses on the little stone ledge behind our coal sheds with the tray between us. We 'podded' the peas, carefully discarding the ones with maggots in. There were inevitably a number of 'bad' peas before the use of pesticides, and shelling had to be done carefully – but speedily, because we *tried* to get to church on time. In the winter we trudged through the snow in our boots, or battled through heavy rain with umbrellas; 'Auntie' wore her galoshes. Our attendance was very regular and nothing stopped us. Like everything in those days, one didn't give in to bombs, weather, headaches or colds.

A church member accompanied the hymns on an old American harmonium. The organist had to push the pedals vigorously with his feet to keep up the power, pressing the swell at each side with his knees to increase the volume when appropriate, while playing the two-manual keyboard and manipulating the various stops. It was good exercise for the calves and thighs, but the sound produced was not in the least beautiful or inspirational. The organists did their best, but none were particularly gifted, and the instrument produced rather a wheezy, droning sound that did nothing to aid the quality of the hearty harmonic - but slow - congregational singing. (Some years later I became one of these organists and I am sure that my efforts at producing a good accompaniment were no better than others, as I struggled with the bellows, the foot swell, the manual and the various organ stops.) One hymn was usually chosen that was especially suitable for the younger members of the congregation.

In order to follow the Scripture reading we had to find the right place in our Bibles. Page numbers were not announced, only the name of the Book and the number of the chapter were given. No Bibles were provided. Everyone carried their own Bible to church and Sunday School, and all the children followed the reading as attentively as the adults, intently fingering each line.

There was a 'children's talk' before the adult sermon, but all the boys and girls (there were not many boys), stayed in the building for the entire service, sitting quietly in the front rows. I can remember passing the time during the sermon silently turning the pages of my Bible, searching for the rose petals I had picked from the garden and pressed between its pages. The fine paper had a delicate, dried-rose scent as I carefully turned over the pages. From time to time I discreetly exchanged a pressed petal or flower with a friend. Illustrated Bible texts on small cards were given out in Sunday School each week. We tucked the extra special ones between the pages of our Bibles and searched these out to look at, learn the text, or reposition them. We occasionally peeped at each other's floral text cards or bookmarks. Class teachers in Sunday School awarded attractive bookmarks with a verse from the Bible printed on the front and these were carefully placed in our Bibles and looked at with pride. I also had coloured pictures of some of the Bible stories in my illustrated

Authorised Version of the Bible to ponder on. All these unobtrusive activities helped to pass the time during the long sermon. I am sure that although I was not listening very closely, or understanding very deeply, I absorbed a lot of the solid Christian teaching that was expounded during the sermon. I became familiar with many of the Bible stories, characters and parables from the sermons, my Bible pictures, and little texts, as well as the lessons I received from my Sunday School teachers.

'Auntie', Rose and I hurried home immediately after the service was over. There was no socialising or coffee following the morning service in those days. I recall very little in the way of general conversation after church either, and everyone sat in silence before the service commenced. (Perhaps a little more quiet contemplation before some services would not come amiss today.) After our walk home from church, the final cooking of the vegetables was done and our Sunday dinner was served. It seemed that as soon as Sunday dinner had been eaten, and the washing up completed, it was time for Rose and me to walk all the way back again for afternoon Sunday School (Bible Class for Rose after her fourteenth birthday). I liked going to Sunday School. After the opening hymn and an extempore prayer (which was also quite lengthy) we sang a number of short rousing choruses before our Bible story and lesson time. I was always eager to choose a chorus, and hoped that the Sunday School Superintendent would sometimes select me from the mass of waving hands of children who were keen to sing their favourite chorus from the C.S.S.M. Chorus Book. (We called it 'Sizzum Choruses', but the initials stood for Children's Special Service Mission, the Christian organisation that began children's beach services and activities at holiday resorts so long ago.)

If I was asked to choose a chorus and had to call out the number, I felt a bit embarrassed at the sound of my voice, but also very pleased that my hand had been noticed waving in the air. We all sang heartily, stamped our feet, clapped our hands and used hands and arms to illustrate the words where appropriate in many of the action choruses. There was little else in the way of physical activity or child participation in Sunday School. I still recall the words and tunes of many of these choruses, could sing them today, and also relate number and some of the words. (Number. 330 - "Be steadfast, unmovable, by faith stand your ground...." is one of many that are still remembered.) Quite a lot of these short songs were chosen, so there were many satisfied boys and girls. How easy it is to recall these songs of long ago, but how difficult it seems to be to remember the words and tunes of some present day worship songs!

After the opening hymn, prayer, choruses and notices, another hymn was sung before we dragged our chairs noisily across the bare boards to form little groups. Circles of about eight children gathered around each teacher, with the boys' classes ranged down the left side of the hall and the girls on the right. The collection was taken and we all put our pennies into the bag that was handed round while the register was taken. During those War years over a hundred children attended each week, many from the nearby council estate, and everyone was given their little illustrated text card as a reward for going to Sunday School. We were encouraged to learn a Bible verse at home relating to the lesson we had heard, and the following week each child recited the verse in turn. When ten weeks' verses had been memorised, a decorative bookmark was given which was proudly placed inside the owner's Bible. Those children who were uncertain about their verse had a chance to polish it up by hearing it recited by the more confident.

A Bible passage was then read around the ring of seated children, with everyone reading a verse in turn. A few girls in my class at Sunday School had difficulty in reading their verse fluently. Not everybody found learning to read easy, but no mothers were allowed in Primary School classrooms in those days to listen to small reading groups; there were no classroom assistants and no special needs teachers. Dyslexia had not been identified and we had all been through a period of broken education. Few families owned many - or any - books, so suitable reading material was not easily available for children at home, unless they lived within walking distance of a Library. All these factors may account for some of the hesitant reading in my Sunday School class, although I don't recall any children in my day school class having reading difficulties. Reading a verse or two in small print, however, from the Authorised Version of the Bible was a very different matter from understanding the words in a graded primer from a reading scheme.

We sat attentively in our groups for the 'reading' and this was followed by the 'lesson'. First of all our teachers retold the Bible story simply and then taught us the lesson they had prepared which related to the particular passage. The emphasis was on listening and learning rather than doing, and I have remembered so many of these Bible stories. Nobody had heard of the old Chinese proverb "I do and I understand", there was no activity time - in fact there was no room for any activity, as we were all grouped very closely together. The teachers spoke fairly quietly in order not to disturb the adjacent group, and there was a subdued hum of noise throughout the hall as they tried to get their lesson across to their pupils in a quiet undertone. Any fidgeting of legs, twiddling of fingers, or whispered chattering was more irritating, and any noise was much magnified in the congestion caused by the closeness of each circle of children. It must have tried the patience of those dedicated adults who gave up their Sunday afternoons week after week to teach in Sunday School. They all had to walk to the church (or use the very infrequent Sunday bus services), had been to the morning service, and would be back in church again in the evening.

One year our Sunday School Superintendent announced a competition to encourage us to learn from memory the names of all the sixty-six books in the Bible. I was very proud to be the winner of this competition, and received a maroon, Moroccan-leather-bound 'Golden Bells' hymnbook, inscribed in beautiful copperplate handwriting on the flyleaf by a beloved Sunday School teacher, Mrs. Fortnam. I was the first person in the Sunday School to recite in correct order the names of the sixty-six books of the Old and New Testament correctly. I have not forgotten them. Nowadays, the page number of the Bible reading is usually announced to the congregation in a church service before the reading, as well as the name of the Book and the number of the chapter. When I was young it was a great help to be able to find the right place quickly, especially if the reading was taken from one of the Minor Prophets! There was a pause before the reading began, which was filled with the sound of rustling pages as everybody hastened to find the appropriate passage.

During the summer many of the girls wore beautiful straw hats to Sunday School. They were made in various shades of cream and beige, woven in different ways to give an assortment of attractive textures. The hats had wide brims to shade our faces from the sun, with garlands of artificial flowers around them, and a coloured ribbon hung down the back. They were individual in style, and as I recall them now, they were really quite charming. (I hope samples of them can still be seen in local museums somewhere in England.) Even on the hottest of Sundays Rose and I wore our hats and net gloves, and I never dreamed of protesting about wearing both a hat and gloves to church or Sunday School!

When I consider the restrictions in clothing at that time I am astonished to realise that I still wore 'best' dresses and coats for Sundays and special days. I wonder whether hats and gloves were exempt from the wartime clothes rationing that prevented any extravagance of design or attempt at manufacturing frivolous clothing. Hats, however, were not considered 'frivolous'; they were part of school uniform and were essential for ladies' and girls' church attendance. Ladies always wore a hat or a headscarf when they went out, even when going shopping, and some made a fashionable headwear of the turban that had to be worn by factory workers. Men wore hats to work and to church, but were careful to show reverence and respect by removing them at the church door. It was, and still is, considered irreverent and inappropriate for men to have their head covered in a church. Girls wore velour hats, and boys wore caps to school. Did one have to part with precious coupons in order to buy a hat?

When I was old enough to ride my bicycle to Sunday School, I still had to wear a flower-trimmed straw hat in summer - with much difficulty if it was a windy day - and my cream net gloves. It was replaced with a black velour school uniform hat in the winter; both hats had elastic under the chin to help to retain them on my head. My father gave me a pair of fur-backed gloves for my Christmas present one year and I remember that Rose had similar fur-backed gloves from her mother – they were probably made from rabbit skin. They were very cosy and comfortable in the cold weather and we often put them on in church during the sermon to keep our hands warm. A big, black, solid-fuel stove took up quite a lot of room on one side of the hall, producing very inadequate heating for the whole building. The slight increase in temperature it produced was insufficient to warm the whole building, and everyone kept their outdoor coats on during the cold weather.

After some time our housekeeper persuaded my father to come to church. I don't remember my parents ever attending church, but perhaps my father decided he would prefer to accompany us on Sunday evenings rather than spend a solitary time at home on his own. I am not sure that he was ever at ease with the service. The American pedal organ was not well played, some of the congregation dragged the singing and the sermon was over-long, very 'sound', but rather 'heavy', although we did have some very good preachers. I was about eleven when my father joined us on our weekly Sunday evening walk and by then I was going to and from church three times on Sundays. 'Auntie', Rose and I went in the morning, Rose and I were back again in the afternoon and all four of us would step it out in the evening. It was such a rush to fit in our meals between all this to-ing and fro-ing. Sundays seemed to consist solely of walking, services, Sunday School, a quick dinner and tea with preparation of the meals and the subsequent washing up in between. At the time it seemed quite normal. Walking to the church and back again three times a day meant that Rose and I walked well over six miles every Sunday. I exchanged most of the walking for pedalling after I had been given a bike, but it was not really a 'Day of rest'! By about 8.30 in the evening we could say that the rest of the day was free time.

Washing up the dishes after our Sunday dinner was not a pleasant task before detergents appeared. A handful of washing soda was put in the water; with perhaps a sprinkle of the Lux soap flakes or Rinso soap powder that was supposed to be used for washing clothes. Saucepans and baking tins were scoured with Vim. The boiler was not lit in the daytime during the summer because it made the kitchen too hot, and we also needed to save fuel, so the kettle and a saucepan of water were heated on the gas stove. The sink and washing up bowl were very greasy at the end of washing the pans and dishes after our Sunday dinner. 'Auntie' washed up and Rose and I were expected to do the drying. My father took no part in this operation. It was considered women's work in those days. 'Auntie's' hands grew very rough and dry, and when my father and I visited my Uncle Connell he occasionally gave us a small bottle of glycerine to take back to 'Auntie', which she massaged into her hands to try soften her skin.

Sunday tea in summertime often included freshly washed lettuce leaves from the garden, which we dipped into a little sugar and vinegar at the side of our plate and ate with bread and butter. I can remember my reluctance to drink my cup of very hot tea after walking home from Sunday School in the heat of the afternoon and being told that the hot tea would cool me down, as it opened the pores! Shipham's sardine and tomato fish paste replaced the lettuce in wintertime and was nearly always followed by one of 'Auntie's home-made Victoria sponges. As I look back now, I feel that Sunday was not my favourite day of the week.

One summer's afternoon Rose and I played truant from Sunday School and Bible Class. We left home on our bicycles at our usual time, but instead of cycling to the church, we made our way to the large Kenton Recreation Ground with its tennis courts, paddling pool, cricket pitches and plenty of open space. We laid our bikes on the ground, pulled off our hats and horrid net gloves and spent the afternoon sunbathing on the grass. Neither of us owned a watch, so we had no idea of the passage of time. We soon grew worried that if we stayed too long at the park we would arrive home later than our normal hour and be found out. We did not really enjoy our little escapade, as we were trying to gauge the time during the entire afternoon and were unable to relax on the grass or revel in our brief freedom. We had no word of reproof when we arrived home. I never knew whether we had been suspected of truanting, or whether all the adults - teachers and parents - concerned had guessed about our prank, but said nothing, in the knowledge (or hope) that we were not really naughty girls (or were we?) and would return to the fold. Perhaps our little escapade had not even been suspected. I never had the inclination to play truant again. The problem of assessing when it was time to go home was much greater than the excitement of our small adventure.

Rose and I got up to another bit of mischief while walking home one summer evening. We hurried on ahead of our respective parents, saying that we walked a lot faster than they did. As soon as they were out of sight we suddenly cut down a side road and played 'Knock Down Ginger'; banging on the door knocker of a house, then running away as fast as we could before bobbing down behind the privet hedge of another house further down the road. Such 'unseemly' behaviour! What a nuisance we must have been on a quiet Sunday evening. We were not caught out, but the excitement made our hearts thump as we squatted on the pavement in the shelter of the hedge until the bemused householder went back inside his house, shut the door, and we knew we were undetected and safe. I don't think our parents ever knew what we got up to during our supposedly sedate walk home that evening. They just wanted to get home in time to listen to 'Sunday Half Hour' on the radio, the 'Palm Court Orchestra' and the classic serial play.

Our Sunday School Anniversaries were very important occasions and we looked forward to these annual events with much anticipation. They always occurred in the summer and seemed to coincide with the period when the roses were at their best. Everyone - teachers, pupils, parents, other members of the congregation and the visiting preacher - wore a rose in his buttonhole on this day, or had one pinned to her dress. Early in the morning Rose and I searched the garden for the nicest rosebuds we could find in the rather sparsely filled flowerbeds. The Sunday school children had been rehearsing for some weeks, coming along to the church after school for an hour's practice of the new or special hymns and songs that we were to sing on Anniversary Day. We rehearsed these special songs to the satisfaction of our very particular choir-mistress, who was also the Sunday School pianist and one of the teachers (the very one who years later became my mother-in-law). I remember one of the hymns began with the words 'Pansies, lilies, roses, flowers of every hue'.

A special preacher was invited to take the services on this day, one who was particularly good at giving children's addresses. During the service the Sunday School 'choir' sang the songs they had practised with joy and enthusiasm. We wore our 'best' clothes, our buttonholes were securely pinned on, our hair freshly washed and curled and everyone was spruced up. The Anniversary day often ended with the hymn, 'Summer suns are glowing, Over land and sea; Happy light is flowing, Bountiful and free'. Anniversaries were very enjoyable and memorable occasions. Despite the gloom and anxiety of wartime, I believe we were happy; we felt free and were not perturbed by, or even aware of, the restrictions in our lives.

Harvest Festivals were also grand occasions. The small building that was our church was decorated with produce and flowers that had been given quite sacrificially from the gardens and allotments, larders and store cupboards of practically everyone in the congregation. Trestle tables were set up at the front of the church and covered with white cloths. Then Mrs. Hull and other ladies in the church arranged the baskets of garden-produced fruit, bunches of home grown carrots, piles of potatoes, onions, large marrows, cabbages and other vegetables that had been brought along. A piece of coal was always displayed, together with some tinned produce and vases of garden flowers. In the middle of the whole array was a large loaf of bread especially made by the local baker. We were indeed thankful for the food we had to eat and that our needs were supplied, and we sang the traditional harvest hymns with enthusiasm and real gratitude to God. All this display had to be dismantled after the evening service,. The produce was distributed to needy people in the church and the nearby Council Estate and the rest was taken to the cottage hospital in Harrow. The trestle tables were then taken down and stored away.

The 'Hut' was only hired and was used during the week as part of the premises of a small, private, preparatory School. All the chairs had to be set out before the morning service, rearranged into circles during our afternoon Sunday School, then put back into rows for the evening service, and finally stacked away again every Sunday evening. The hymnbooks and chorus books were locked up in 'our' cupboard and the floor swept ready for its different Monday morning use. How dedicated were the members of this little congregation and what sacrifices they made in time, money and perhaps personal relationships, to keep their little church going. The old wooden hall and the little Prep. School were demolished long ago, but a new permanent church was built in the late l950s, and paid for by the members, on land they had bought when Kenton College closed.

Our housekeeper was friendly with a family at church and their daughter Janet and I became 'Sunday friends'. It was with her that I sometimes exchanged my pressed rose petals and compared the beauty, size or quality of our little text cards, as we sat quietly through the morning service. Her father was the Sunday School Superintendent. Occasionally our family was invited to Sunday tea with Mr. and Mrs. Hull.

We all sat around their wartime dining table, which was a reinforced metal Morrison Air Raid shelter. This was larger than a domestic dining table and was used during the air raids for the family to take shelter beneath. It was named after Herbert Morrison, who was a member of the Cabinet, Home Secretary and Minister of Home Security.

'Auntie' always took a little bit of our butter ration wrapped in greaseproof paper on these tea-time visits, together with a small screw of paper containing a little tea, and a little bag of sugar to help replace that which had been used in the baking of cakes. We didn't want to deplete our friends' rations. Going out to tea in someone else's home was quite a rare occurrence in those times. Bouquets of flowers, boxes of chocolates, or bottles of wine were not the kinds of 'thank you for having me' gifts that were presented then, but a contribution to one's hosts' food allowances! Janet's 'Nanna' was sometimes present, but I never wondered why I didn't have a grandma, nor did I wonder why Mr. and Mrs. Hull and their daughter never came to tea at our house. I can't recall us ever having visitors to tea when I was young.

My friendship with Janet developed as we grew older. Although she was only two years younger, when you are ten or eleven, someone aged eight or nine seemed a very little girl. The age difference diminished a few years later when we played tennis together and after we had grown up it had quite lost any significance. She was a bridesmaid at my wedding years later and we are still in touch with each other.

Chapter Ten

HARD TIMES

Shortages of various necessities (such as toilet rolls!), queues for food, and the drudgery of housework made daily life quite hard for everyone. Children were expected to help with the household duties, and I soon began to appreciate the problems our housekeeper had in providing nourishing meals, together with the difficulties entailed in keeping us all warm and well clothed. Food rationing came into force in 1940 and was not totally abolished until June 1954. I had to take my ration book with me on my honeymoon in 1952, still registered in my maiden name, much to my embarrassment at the time. After the War ended in 1945, food became even more scarce because of the desperate needs in the shattered countries of war-torn Europe. Bread was not rationed during the whole of the War, but in 1946 coupons were required to buy this staple food.

The basic rations for each person every week were: 2oz butter (50g); 2oz cheese (50g) - sometimes rising to 4 or even 8oz; 4oz margarine (125g); 2oz lard (50g); 8oz sugar (250g); 2oz tea (50g); 4oz bacon (125g); ½ pint milk per day for children (adult allowance varied between ¼ and ½ pint per day); 1lb. jam or marmalade every 8 weeks; 1s. 2d-worth of meat (about 6p), and 1 egg (when available).

The sugar ration appears to have been a very generous allowance and I am sure I don't use 500g of sugar a week nowadays, but a 'sweet tooth' was very common - even sixty years ago. Sugar consumption was perhaps more obvious then, with fewer highly sweetened, ready-made convenience foods containing 'hidden sugar' to tempt the housewife. Most people took sugar in their tea and sprinkled it on corn flakes or porridge. Much more cooking was done at home; baking cakes, bottling fruit, making jam, pickles and chutneys. Sweets and chocolates and soft drinks were only occasional treats.

Consumers were allowed to use their meat ration in whatever way they wished from what was available at the local butcher's shop. If the cheaper cuts of meat were chosen the family could have a little more in quantity. Everyone had to be registered with a butcher and a grocer and had to purchase their rations from those particular shops. Vegetables were not rationed and could be bought at any greengrocer's shop.

'Auntie' used to cut our weekly 8oz. block of butter into four equal portions, and these were placed on two dishes, one for her and Rose, and the other for my father and me. Each little 2oz piece of butter had our initial inscribed on it with a knife, and at mealtimes we each buttered our own bread, making sure that we used our personal allowance, re-carving our initial if we had scraped it off as we used our portion of butter. It ensured that we all had our fair share, and 'P' and 'S' appeared on the small pieces of butter on my father's and my dish. The little blocks of butter did not go far; as the week wore on our initials became less and less distinguishable as each portion diminished in size. We had to spread hard Stork margarine on our bread before our next allocation of butter was due! Vegetable oils were not obtainable then and lard or meat dripping was used for frying. 'Auntie' did not eat pork or any pork derived food, and for a long time the coupons for our lard ration was left untouched. We never had pork meat and I cannot remember whether my father and I ever had bacon or ham, but believe that this part of our food allowance was also unclaimed.

George, our friendly milkman, made his daily round with his horse and cart. He placed our one-and-a-half pints of milk on our doorstep every morning, while 'Queenie', the horse, walked at a leisurely pace, pausing for George to make his small deliveries. 'Queenie' seemed to sense when it was time for her to 'walk on' a few steps before George had even begun to cross the road. There was no refrigeration on his cart, or any means of keeping the crates of milk cool in hot weather, and our milk was often tepid by the time it reached our house in the summer, even though George always placed the milk in the more shaded corner of our porch.

Although I lived in a developing suburb, Kenton Lane Farm was less than half a mile away from my home. I sometimes walked up the road to the farmyard in the holidays and stood outside the gate leading to the milking-parlour while the cows were being milked. I had to stand at a distance to watch the empty bottles chugging around the conveyor belt as they were washed and sterilised. J. H. Brazier's was a family dairy farm, and cattle grazed in some fields nearby, but I didn't know then that they had much more land a few miles away in Stanmore. The farmhouse in Kenton Lane is still lived in by one of the Brazier family at the time I write, and the large dairy business is thriving in Oxhey, on the rural outskirts of Watford, supplying milk to local residents and further afield.

Despite our restricted diet there didn't appear to be much illness in our family or in the community, and there were never many absentees from school. 'Auntie' often had bad backache and she sometimes sat on a chair, leaning over the kitchen table with her head on her arms while Rose massaged her back and neck, to the accompaniment of 'oohs' and 'aahs' when extra tender areas were rubbed. Both Rose and her mother sometimes had migraine headaches; my father and I had frequent catarrhal colds. A visit to the doctor was a rare experience in my childhood, but when I did see him I found the waiting room was drab and dull with a row of old dining chairs lining the walls. There was nothing to read and certainly no toys to amuse the children. One sat patiently waiting (is that why we are called 'patients'?) for one's turn to come into his equally dull, shabby and sombre surgery. There was no appointment system, no receptionist, no nurses or ancillary staff, just the local doctor in his back room surgery, usually held in his own home.

Visits to the dentist were equally infrequent. Regular check-ups were unknown and I only sat in the dentist's chair once or twice in my childhood, when I had been suffering from toothache. The need for a filling, or more likely, the extraction of a tooth, was not at all like the quite pleasant visit to one's dentist nowadays.

I came home for my mid-day meal as school dinners were not available in Primary School then. 'Auntie' often baked apples in the oven for our pudding with some of the fruit that had been stored in the garage from our apple trees. I have a strong memory of struggling to eat a rather sour, but very hot, baked apple for my 'afters'. I sometimes scalded the inside of my mouth as I swallowed it, trying to get it finished before rushing back to school in time for afternoon registration.

Yoghurt appeared later on in the War and could be bought in little pots at the Express Dairy. It was so sour and acidic that it made me shudder as I tried to eat it. Children were expected to eat whatever food was put in front of them, and although I found it so difficult to swallow that sour, unsweetened, strong yoghurt and to eat the very hot apple, I would not dream of refusing to eat something I didn't like! Sweetened or fruit yoghurts were not introduced until many years after the War ended. There were few convenience foods in the shops, although when large, individual jam tarts were spotted on the counter of the Express Dairy shop, a selection of them were bought for our pudding. We carefully considered who would have the one with raspberry jam, or blackcurrant jam, or the one filled with synthetic lemon curd.

In most towns there was what was called a British Restaurant, which provided a very basic meal at a reasonable price. It was eagerly patronised by the elderly, or those living alone, who although they had the same allocation of food as everyone else had greater difficulty in producing a main meal for themselves each day. Meals were available for employees in factory canteens and there were some restaurants in big towns and cities, but there were no cafes in my locality - only the fish and chip shop! How different from today, when almost every other shop in the High Street seems to be a restaurant or food outlet of some kind.

It was a difficult task trying to provide adequate meals every day of the week from our rations, but our housekeeper managed to concoct some tasty dinners from the food available. She sometimes made a cheese batter pudding, which came out of the oven with a lovely crispy top. We didn't consider it to be a vegetarian dish at the time and knew nothing about a vegetarian life style, but we often had what we called 'meatless meals'. We might have a plate of cooked vegetables - carrots, parsnips, potato and cabbage - for our dinner, smothered with a cheese sauce, which was very tasty and satisfying. I now realise that it was very nourishing too, but little was known about food values, vitamins, or protein requirements then. A plateful of food for dinner was the main desire, but I think we were possibly better nourished than many today. When the milk yield was high, more cheese was available; the cheese ration was sometimes increased, which helped to eke out our meagre meat ration. We ate corned beef in our house, but never had Spam or liver, due to our housekeeper's aversion to any kind of pork or offal. Liver was not rationed and would have made a useful protein meal.

Fish was sometimes of very dubious quality and of doubtful freshness. The fishmonger had his display of so-called fresh fish arrayed outside his fried fish shop, but during the summer months we often had our doubts as to its freshness. At times there was a strong smell of ammonia surrounding the shop; we believed he washed his leftover fish in ammonia or chlorine and then sold it the following day. Sometimes the fried fish had a faint, unpleasant ammonia taste - one was safer with the chips! Nevertheless, if we happened to buy fish and chips for dinner on one of his 'good' days, when the fish was fresh, it made a useful, off ration, meal. Fish and chips were always wrapped in newspaper and we sometimes took our spare newspapers to the fish shop or the butcher's to help their supply of wrapping paper.

After the War my friends and I sometimes hung around the fish and chip shop in the evenings. We bought 'two-pennyworth of chips', or if we were hard up we could buy 'one-pennyworth of chibbles'. We didn't go 'clubbing' or 'partying' in my youth. We would not dream of congregating around the pub with the possible intention of under-age drinking, buying or taking drugs, being involved in hooliganism, or a possible victim of violence, mugging, rape or murder. No one seemed aggressive, insulting or abusive. World War was surrounding us and daily life was tough, but life in our society was more than relatively peaceful. Why has that life disappeared?

I often had to help with the shopping and can vividly remember the queues, the unexpected arrival of a scarce commodity, the occasional appearance of tinned fruit, or tins of Australian 'IXL' melon and ginger jam placed inconspicuously on the top shelf of our local Express Dairy shop. Observant customers - sometimes *me* - soon spotted them and they remained on display for a very short while before word got around, and eager housewives snapped them up. We thought melon and ginger jam was most unusual, and it was a real change from ordinary fare. We were also able to buy 'IXL' peach jam from time to time, which contained large chunks of fruit, and it was so much better than the jars of jam normally available with the 'points' at the back of our ration books. Jam was a much more essential commodity than it is today and our tea would frequently consist of bread and butter (or margarine) and jam – homemade if we were lucky. We were occasionally able to buy small tins of blackcurrant puree from the chemist's shop. It was rich in vitamin C and I think this was why the chemist, but not the grocer, sold this product. It was very nutritious and a real fruity treat.

My father was paid each week in cash, as was the majority of the lower middle-class population in those days. I never knew how much he gave 'Auntie' for her wages each Friday evening, but I know that she was given £2 each week for housekeeping money. This had to pay for food for us all and cover other minor household expenses for the following week. When I was considered old enough I did the weekend shopping on Saturdays. Most of my Saturday morning seemed to be taken up with completing this task, as there were queues at nearly all the shops in our nearby parade. The first shop I came to was the Victoria Wine Company, the local 'off-licence' which only opened for a few hours each day at unusual hours. It never seemed to be open or to have any customers when I passed by and I never went inside. The next shop was Wincups, the newsagent, tobacconist and sweet shop. It had a counter at the back that served as the local Post Office. This was followed by Mr. Marchant's ironmonger's shop. Mr. Marchant lived in Kenton Lane and we occasionally saw him walking home from his shop in the evening.

The Manageress of the Express Dairy was a severe-looking lady who wore her hair in two plaits wound around each side of her head like earphones or two Chelsea buns. We thought they covered her ears, and were always curious to know how she was able to hear what her customers asked for. We called her the 'bun lady' - but not to her face. Self-service was unthought-of and I am sure our rather peremptory but efficient Express Dairy 'bun lady' would have totally disapproved of any of her customers serving themselves. There was rarely a queue at her shop and she didn't appear to have a very wide range of food. Jackman's, the greengrocer's, was still there and owned by the same family when I last saw it, and looked much as I remembered it, with the potatoes, carrots and green vegetables in exactly the same compartments as when I was young.

Mr. Cox owned the butcher's shop, but both Mr. Cox and his shop have now long since departed. The floor of his shop was covered with wood shavings that were swept up each evening and replaced with fresh ones before he opened the following day. Mr. Cox was a big, fat man with a cheerful red face, who wrapped our little joints of meat or stewing lamb in newspaper. Mr. Selby also lived nearby in Kenton Lane and owned the chemist's shop; its dark mahogany counter and glass cabinets displaying large jars filled with bright but unknown liquid, gave the shop a sombre, serious, mysterious impression. Mr. Selby died long ago, but his business continued under the same name for many years. It is still a pharmacy, but now with a new owner and the glass jars and important-looking cabinets have disappeared. Bread was baked daily on the premises at the baker's shop. There was a hairdresser's and an inadequately stocked draper's shop, with very few items on the shelves, and window dressing that would be considered 'minimalist' today. The lady who owned it must have had a hard time keeping her shop going through the War. (My father would have had a similar difficulties if he had retained the ownership of his little menswear' shop.)

Whyborn's the 'wireless shop' did a variety of simple electrical repairs and was where one could buy small electrical items, torches (essential for getting around in the dark) and batteries. Mr. Whyborn also recharged the accumulators in his customers' wireless sets from time to time. Next to his shop was the shoe repairer, where the smell of leather permeated the air inside and outside the shop. The roar and clattering of the machinery, which was used to repair our shoes, made it necessary to shout in order to be heard. Shoes frequently needed mending; heels wore down quickly, soles soon grew thin and holes appeared, because everybody walked so much. My father had a shoe last (a foot-shaped metal block used for repairing shoes) and did most of our shoe repairs at home, so I rarely had to suffer the din and the strong smell of leather in this shop.

Peark's was another grocer's shop at the far end of our Parade. It was much smaller than Sainsbury's in Kenton High Street, but it also had its separate dairy and grocery counters and customers had to queue at both counters for their different purchases. The Assistant at the dairy counter was kept busy gauging the correct cheese allowance before slicing it off the large round cheese with a wire cutter. Sometimes we had to have a cut off the block of 'processed' cheese. We were not used to processed food in those days! She also had to cut and shape a lump of butter with her wooden butter patters to the exact weight for each family's weekly allowance. She marked each ration card, indicating that the week's allocation had been taken. The Assistant on the grocery counter cut out the 'points' coupons when any of the additional limited items, such as corn flakes, baked beans, sardines or the rare tin of salmon, were available. (We had never heard of fresh salmon.) Calculations for purchases were made mentally, the cash taken from the customer and accurate change given by each Assistant. They had many jobs to do behind the counter. It is not surprising that we waited a long time before we were served.

On one occasion our housekeeper was being served at the dairy counter and as usual had refused our ration of lard (which of course was made from pork), when the customer behind her quietly whispered into her ear, "If you buy your lard ration, I will exchange it for 8oz of my margarine ration. My family like a lot of fried food and I could do with some more cooking fat." So from then on 'Auntie' bought our 2oz. per person lard ration each week and I used to walk or cycle to a house some way away from our home with the packet of lard and come back with an 8oz block of margarine. 'Auntie' had managed to acquire an extra supply of margarine, which she used for making her pastry as well as our cakes. We were all well pleased that we now had our full allowance of fat to use during those lean years.

The last shop in our parade, called 'Reader's, was a subscription lending Library. The rear wall of the shop was lined with shelves of rather tired-looking books and it also stocked minor stationery items, a few sweets and cigarettes. As I never used its Library service I didn't appreciate the significance of the name 'Readers' for many years. The arrival of the new public Library must have produced much competition for the owner of this shop. No doubt he had his small clientele who were prepared to pay for the romantic fiction or thrillers they wanted to borrow, instead of making a long walk for a better selection of books in the Library. It always looked a very dull shop to me.

We didn't have far to go for all our daily needs, and I knew many of the shop Assistants, some of them by name. 'Auntie' usually bought the grocery rations at Pearks at the beginning of the week, but I often had to queue for a long time outside the butcher's, the baker's and especially the greengrocer's on Saturday mornings. The customers waited patiently outside Jackman's, stamping their cold feet on the pavement in the winter, occasionally shuffling forward a few steps before another long wait. At last another move forward occurred, followed by yet another long pause before we moved again slowly towards the shop window. Time seemed to drag even more slowly the nearer one got to the entrance, but eventually I was inside and served at last.

The queue at the greengrocer's was always the longest, both in time and in distance. It often stretched along the length of the shop-front and then snaked across the wide pavement to the road and sometimes curled back on itself at the edge of the pavement. There was only one greengrocer's shop for a very large community and every customer had to have her purchases weighed up individually; there were no pre-packed goods and no pre-washed vegetables either. They all had their layer of dirt and chunks of hard clay were sometimes still attached to the potatoes, which cost 6d. (5p) for 7lb. The baker's queue was also very long, but it moved a bit faster as customers didn't require so many different items of food.

One Saturday morning a pound note was put into the 'housekeeping purse' and I set off with a large basket and a shopping list to do the weekend shopping. I had nearly finished my round of purchases when I discovered that I hadn't enough money left in the purse to complete the shopping. I thought I must have dropped a ten-shilling note somewhere. Ten shillings was an enormous amount for me to lose and I had no idea of how or where I could have dropped it. I went back to all the shops, asked several people if they had seen my money, but nobody knew anything about it. I was so worried. I didn't have the courage to go home and confess that I had lost a quarter of the entire week's housekeeping allowance. I knew my father was very short of money and I sat down on a seat outside Wincups feeling very worried, and not knowing what else to do.

After a while a lady came up and asked me what the matter was. I told her what had happened and that I did not dare to go back home. She was very kind, tried to reassure me and offered to walk home with me. She explained to our housekeeper that she had found me looking anxious and upset, and how I had told her my story. I understood only too well the seriousness of what had happened and felt ashamed of myself for being so irresponsible. I can't remember the immediate consequences, but think that 'Auntie', and my father, when he came home from work in the evening, understood that I had not meant to be careless, but they were both worried at the loss of the cash. It didn't enter our thoughts - or certainly not mine - that the money might have been stolen from me.

Nowadays we are more aware of the possibility of petty thieves in busy shopping areas, ready to prey on a child or the elderly. Maybe someone was looking out for and taking advantage of a young shopper. We did not think of dishonesty in our streets and nobody seemed to fear that they might be robbed in the district where I lived. The fear of crime was not in people's minds then – although I now know that looting occurred on bombsites, and a 'black market' was active in many parts of the country. We went out of our houses without locking our back doors, nor felt it necessary to keep the side gate bolted. I guess that nobody had very much that was worth stealing, but I believe I grew up in a more honest society.

I had either carelessly dropped the ten shilling note, or someone had accidentally omitted to give me all my 'change'; it could not have been deliberately stolen. Somebody found the ten-shilling note on the pavement and had picked it up, or one of the shops found they had made ten shillings extra profit when they cashed up at the end of the day. We were the ones who had to go a bit short of food for the rest of that week. One begins to realise the truth of the saying, 'Living from hand to mouth' when considering the (not so distant) past.

When time dragged on a dreary winter's afternoon in the school holidays, my friends and I sometimes 'hung around' in Wincups. We often didn't know how to amuse ourselves, so we spent a long time in the sweet shop, chatting to the Assistant while making up our minds - and no doubt changing them. Should we buy a few aniseed balls, a sherbet dab, a liquorice 'bootlace', a liquorice wheel with a sweet in the middle, a bag of 'love hearts', some sherbet lemons, pear drops or some other sweet treat? Sweet rationing was introduced in 1942, but I have no recollection of handing over any coupons for these children's goodies, (or 'baddies', as many of these highly coloured and artificially flavoured sweets must have been for our teeth). Perhaps they disappeared with the arrival of the sweet ration? The official allowance was 12oz. (325g) per person a month and as I grew older I think I became more circumspect in my choice of sweets - or the selection became more restricted.

My school friends and I were not really concerned about the limitations put on our sweet consumption. We had not been brought up to eat many sweets. We were probably more restricted by the amount of pocket money we received. I think I had three pence a week (just over 1p now) for most of the years I was at primary school, but I was also given a penny for church and Sunday School collections, and my comic was paid for each week. I had had no training in the handling of my own money when I started work at sixteen years of age. This did not seem to affect my ability to look after my personal finances and purchases as an adult, other than possibly making me more cautious in spending on extravagant items. Self-indulgent or excessive spending was impossible for most people who grew up in that period, and old habits die hard. One's 'needs' were more easily satisfied than 'wants'.

Carrots always seemed plentiful, even during the War, and their benefits were often extolled in the Radio Doctor's words of wisdom on the wireless every Tuesday morning after the 8 o'clock news. A recipe was once given for carrot jam! I think 'Auntie' made some and we found it very sweet and rather tasteless, but it provided something to spread on our bread for tea. I sometimes went into the greengrocer's shop before school if I left home with time to spare, and bought a halfpenny carrot – or did it only cost a farthing? Maud, the Assistant, wiped it down her overall before handing the carrot over to me. I paid my small sum of money and went off happily munching my carrot as if it was a sweet. No doubt it was better for me, despite its inadequate cleaning, than the sweets I bought in pre-ration days at Wincups. I must have taken Olwen's saying, advising one to 'Eat a peck of dirt before you die', to heart! I hope I equally remembered the table of weights we had to learn in school, with the line of 'four pecks equal one bushel'.

Mr. Marchant's ironmonger's shop always had a pungent smell, with a blend of paraffin, paint and dog biscuits. He had sacks of grain for those who, like our next-door neighbours, kept a few chickens at the bottom of their back garden, hoping to have some extra eggs. Sacks of straw supplied fresh 'bedding' for those who kept rabbits, and sacks of bone meal, dog biscuits and various other domestic requirements took up most of the rest of the floor space in the shop. There was always a long queue of customers patiently waiting in the limited space beside all these sacks. Customers' requirements were so varied, stock was in so many different places and Mr. Marchant didn't hurry himself. A one-yard brass measure fixed to the back of the worn wooden counter helped him to calculate the length of certain items customers asked for. Seemingly hundreds of tiny boxes of all sizes of loose nails, screws, hooks and other useful oddments were amongst his miscellaneous stock.

Bundles of firewood were neatly piled up beneath the front of the counter, but I didn't know then that my grandfather's livelihood had depended upon firewood! In fact I never thought about a grandfather. I certainly did not know that my mother, whom I now rarely thought about, had sometimes joined her father on his cart when she was a girl, as his horse trotted around the oil shops and ironmongers in south London, selling the firewood that had been chopped and bundled at the bottom of the back yard of her childhood home in Rotherhithe. It was more than thirty years later that my mother told me this, as she reminisced about her childhood. I had no concept of a grandfather, or curiosity about my parents' childhood. I wish I had asked more questions!

We used firewood to help to light the fire at home. Sticks of firewood were carefully laid in our hearth on top of screwed up newspaper; the knobs of coal were arranged on top and a match was lit to the paper. The flames of the burning paper soon ignited the wood, a crackle was heard and hopefully, the coal gradually began to burn and the fire was alight. Sometimes the fire would suddenly die back and a sheet of newspaper had to be held firmly across the front of the fireplace opening, to try to create a strong draught to rekindle the coal. After a few minutes the paper was removed and a great gust of smoke blew up towards the ceiling and a horrible smell filtered through the room. It was a great relief to see the flames had become steady and the coal was beginning to glow. The sound of the flames from the fire and the sight of the coal burning brightly was such a relief we didn't mind the smell. (It was not surprising that our homes got dirty quickly and required such regular cleaning.) The rise in temperature that was eventually felt in the cold room was worth all the effort, but it was rather a dangerous practice.

Our coal ration sometimes consisted of poor quality fuel and often contained a lot of coal dust that didn't burn well. A 'recipe' was given by the Government to encourage the public to make a coal substitute with this dust and turn it into a combustible fuel, but it was not very successful. The hazards and excitements involved in trying to get a room warm are almost forgotten with the efficiency of our time-controlled, temperature-regulated, central heating and artificial gas-flame imitation 'coal' fires, but everyone had an open fire before the post-War era arrived. Fireplaces, hearths, grates and chimneys are rarely seen in newly built houses and no doubt these words will gradually disappear from the vocabulary!

Solid fuel fires produced a lot of ash, which had to be cleaned out from beneath the grates of our living room fire and the kitchen boiler each morning and taken outside. Clinkers, the hard cinders that would not burn up, were also removed. All these essential dirty jobs contributed to the hard work of the housewife. The kitchen boiler was a great comfort though, and we enjoyed sitting around it at odd moments during a cold winter's day, lifting down the front to reveal the glowing coke or anthracite fire behind the bars. But the fire needed stoking regularly from the coke-hod that was kept at the side of the boiler. This had to be replenished twice daily from the coal shed behind the garage, at the end of the path that went half way down the garden. It was not a job any of us desired in snowy or icy weather, but it still had to be filled, as did the coalscuttle for the fire in the living room. We tried to conserve our precious fuel and the fire was not lit until mid-afternoon. There was often much concern during the winter season about the possibility of running out of coal or coke before the coalman delivered the next allocation.

Housework was hard work and done to a regular routine. Monday was traditionally washing day. I can faintly remember seeing the dirty clothes being stuffed into a gas copper by my mother when I was very young. The gas was lit beneath it and the water was brought to the boil. The steamy brew was stirred from time to time with a 'dolly', pushing it up and down and moving the clothes around to help to loosen the dirt. The washing was then rinsed by hand in the big earthenware 'butler' sink before being wrung through a hand-turned mangle that was kept in a corner of the garden. Shirts and pillowcases were starched before being finally wrung and hung up to dry. Washing was a lengthy job and a hard day's work.

'Auntie' found that all the washing for a household of four, as well as the white cotton sheets from four beds, was too much for her, so the clothes' boiler was disposed of and the sheets were sent to the laundry. A large galvanised iron bucket of water replaced the gas boiler and this was filled with water and heaved on to the top of the gas stove early every Monday morning. Soap powder was added and the items of clothing that required more than a wash and a scrub on the scrubbing board in the sink were pushed into the bucket. The gas tap was turned full on and the clothes were left to come to the boil with an occasional stirring and prodding with an old wooden spoon, before the usual rinsing. We didn't have coloured sheets, towels or underwear, and a 'blue bag' was swirled around in the last rinsing water to give the 'whites' a whiter look before the wringing process. There was still a long line of clothes to be hung on the washing-line in our garden.

If an icy wind blew against the wet clothes hanging on the line in the garden in the winter, the washing often froze during the day, and when I came home from school in the afternoon I was sometimes asked to bring it in. I often found everything stiff and unwieldy, and impossible to fold until it had thawed out. Shirts or blouses 'stood up' as if there was a body inside them. On wet days we dried the washing in the kitchen on a line that ran alongside the wall next to our solid fuel boiler. The warmth helped to dry the clothes but the smell of damp clothes was unpleasant when I came home from school. The various garments hanging about made the usually warm, cheery room very dismal, and washing still draped over the line at breakfast the following morning was a miserable beginning to the day.

The linoleum on the kitchen floor plus the red tiles of the scullery were scrubbed once a week. A hard scrubbing brush, bar of Sunlight soap, a bucket of hot water and a floor cloth were needed for this job. When I came home from school on hot summer afternoons I sometimes found 'Auntie' on her hands and knees, looking very weary and over-heated as she came to the end of this energetic task. She spread sheets of newspaper over the scrubbed parts of the floor until it had dried and I had to tiptoe carefully through the kitchen, treading only on the sheets of newspaper. The lino was then finished off with wax Mansion polish and more 'elbow grease' until it gleamed, and the tiles were polished with bright red Cardinal polish to enhance their colour and keep them shiny too.

All the furniture and the lino that surrounded each carpet square in the two living rooms and two main bedrooms, was polished every week. The bathroom and my little bedroom floor were covered with lino and needed the same treatment from time to time. A strip of carpet ran through the hall, with areas of lino at both sides, which also required polishing. The staircase carpet was held in place by wooden stair-rods and this was brushed briskly with a stiff bristle hand brush. We had an elderly, noisy, early model of a Hotpoint vacuum cleaner for the carpets.

What a tremendous amount of energy and hard physical work was required of the housewife before fitted carpets, washing machines and central heating became an accepted part of our daily lives. It's no wonder that children were expected to help with household tasks. Keep Fit classes, the Gym, Health Clubs or 'personal trainers' were not necessary for young women to have aerobic exercise in the early-to-mid-twentieth century. Keeping the house clean burned up many calories, strengthened bones and toughened arm muscles, but was very tiring and time-consuming - hard labour in fact. Home-helps or charladies, as they used to be called, were very scarce in wartime. Most women were doing some kind of war-work as well as their household duties. But our house was kept spotlessly clean.

In between all this housework and shopping, the meals were prepared and baking done. All our cakes and pastry were homemade - with the exception of the Express Dairy's jam tarts and my personal visits to the baker for his Wednesday afternoon doughnuts. On my way home from Senior School I was often drawn irresistibly to the baker's shop by the delicious smell of the freshly baked, sugar-coated doughnuts that were brought straight from the bakery on huge trays and tipped into a large area immediately behind the shop window. The temptation was often too great and one of my pocket-money pennies was spent on a doughnut, oozing with red jam as I bit into it. We were often quite hungry in wartime and longed for a little extra to fill us up. I treated myself on Wednesday afternoons. Girls did not need to worry about dieting in those days!

I often sat at one end of the kitchen table when 'Auntie' was preparing pastry or making a cake. Making a Victoria sponge cake was another energetic process, beating the sugar and margarine round and round the bowl with a fork or a wooden spoon until it was light and creamy, and whisking up the reconstituted dried egg mixture with a hand whisk before adding it to the flour. There was no electric food mixer to do the job in a few seconds, but the cake was always light and, when filled with some homemade plum jam from our Victoria plum tree, it was a real treat for Sunday tea. 'Auntie' often made pastry for a fruit pie to finish off our Sunday dinner during the winter, using one of the jars of golden plums that we had bottled in the summer, or some of the apples that were stored in the garage. I am sure my interest in cookery was generated during the hours I sat and watched her baking activities. I was also waiting to scrape out and eat the remains of the cake mixture from the mixing bowl - or half of it if Rose was around, when a line carefully marked down the centre ensured equal shares for both of us!

'Auntie's elderly widowed mother lived locally and when she became ill she was brought to our house. My father moved downstairs to sleep on the Put-u-up in the living room and she was cared for in his bedroom until she died. She never left her bed after she came to live with us. I recall a very quiet, hushed period around the time of her death. I did not really understand what was happening, but I do remember going into the bedroom and seeing this old lady lying with her eyes closed and her head on the pillows of my father's bed shortly before - or it might have been after - she died. Her funeral cortege left from our home and 'Auntie' was very sad for some time. She was the only daughter and Rose was the only granddaughter. Some of their relatives came to the house for refreshments after the funeral, but I was not really involved. It was the only death I experienced during my childhood, and although it was in my own home I remember very little about it. After her death my father returned to his own bedroom but, sadly, not for very long.

He was still having great difficulty in 'making ends meet'. There was not much business at Meakers; commission on sales was slight and wages in the clothing trade had never been generous. With two mortgages to pay, and providing for the needs of our 'family' of four, paying his housekeeper a wage had become impossible and he thought she would have to leave us. It would have been very difficult for 'Auntie' and her daughter to find alternative accommodation in wartime, so a compromise was reached, and she agreed to remain as housekeeper without any actual wage other than the provision of a home for herself and Rose, together with all their meals. She stayed on with us, but also got a part-time office job. Rose had finished her education, completed a Pitman's secretarial course, had started work, and so could help her mother a little, so the critical period was eased and life continued more or less as before - for a while.

These economies, however, were soon found to be inadequate, and my father found yet another way to meet all our needs; we had a lodger. A lady came to live in what had been my parents' bedroom. This was let as a furnished bed-sitting room and my parents' bedroom suite was retained for the lodger's use. The small gentleman's wardrobe that had been put into my little bedroom was now shared between my father and I. An electric hot plate was bought for the lodger, along with a small folding table, and an easy chair appeared from somewhere. It could not have been a very cosy room to live in, but our lady lodger was relieved to have a roof over her head, as accommodation was so difficult to find. Miss Rich was at work all day and we found she was a very pleasant, quiet little lady. Our paths did not seem to cross very often and sometimes we did not see her for days. Her weekly rent, though small, helped my father to provide the necessities of life for 'Auntie', Rose, himself and me, and to pay the bills. A domestic catastrophe was averted.

Our lodger's life in that room now seems to me to have been very solitary, with only basic necessities. However, she continued to live with us until just before I married in 1952, when my husband-to-be and I were going to share the house with my father. (Her bed-sit then became our living room until after our first son was born. An accommodation crisis is nothing new! Our new furniture and curtains changed the character of the room once again, making it look much more comfortable.)

My father had given up his bedroom and now slept on the Put-u-up downstairs. This was opened out each evening at bedtime and folded away every morning to allow us to use the room during the day. Every night the dining table and chairs were shifted across to a corner of the room, and pushed back again each morning. He had now, in effect, lost his wife, slept on a folding bed in his own house, and had no bedroom, or even a wardrobe of his own in which to keep his clothes. Our lady lodger lived in the main bedroom. Rose and her mother slept in what had been my bedroom, and I had the third single bedroom. My father was without any male companionship and saw very little of his few relatives. He lived in an all female household and had no close friends – in fact, he saw none of the friends he and my mother used to have; difficulties with transport made visiting almost impossible. He accepted all these deprivations without comment or complaint, but I now realise how much he had to put up with as I grew up; how deprived he was; how lonely he must have been.

Although he was a very reserved person who never expressed his thoughts or feelings, I remember him as a cheerful man, often singing, never complaining or moody. He was not demonstrative, and our closest contact, other than a brief goodnight kiss, was when I danced with him to the music of his old records at Christmas time, or when we occasionally had what we called 'mock fights' and wrestled affectionately through the kitchen and along the length of our hall.

Chapter Eleven

WINTER IN WARTIME

We experienced very severe winters in the early nineteen forties with dense, 'pea-soup' fogs, when you could scarcely see a hand in front of you, hard frosts, heavy falls of snow. The house never seemed to be thoroughly heated; the hall and bedrooms were always chilly. Carpet was quite thin and lino was a cold surface - especially to one's feet when stepping out of bed in the morning. Cold houses often meant frozen or burst pipes and there was real hardship if the coal shed became empty.

As I walked to school on wintry mornings I sometimes saw rows of icicles hanging down from the gutters, or a mound of ice bulging from the top of a drainpipe. An icy tongue of frozen water drooped from the base of a down-pipe. A burst pipe was possible if a sudden thaw occurred. Occasionally the water froze in our galvanised iron cold-water tank in the loft. Loft insulation was not common in those days, pipes were not lagged and loft floors or roof timbers were not protected from the weather - but if ever it was needed, insulation was required then. If no water ran when the cold tap was turned on in the morning, or the toilet cistern didn't refill after flushing, we knew we were in trouble. We would have to let the kitchen boiler go out. We couldn't flush the toilet or use any water until either the frozen system had thawed, or the plumber had been called in to mend a burst pipe. Plumbers were not 'central-heating consultants' in those days, but 'burst pipe repairers' who were kept very busy in winter months.

Those bitterly cold winters have not occurred in recent years. Their absence seems to be more than just a swing of the pendulum of changing weather patterns, but a possible indication of global warming. Yet we are better prepared for cold weather in this millennium than in the last, but seemingly ill equipped to cope with the new weather patterns of rainstorms, tornadoes and widespread flooding. I wouldn't like to return to those harsh cold days of my childhood. We had many rainy days, but there was not the fear of our home being inundated with water, local flooding of our roads because of blocked drains, or the greater risk of flooding on a large scale in some areas of the country. Large housing estates were not built on flood plains then.

Our solid fuel boiler provided some warmth in the kitchen during the day. We couldn't spare the fuel to heat a lot of water, and the kitchen boiler was too small to heat sufficient for a family to bathe every day, so we could only have one bath each week, with only a little water in the bath. The public was informed that the King had ordered that nobody was allowed to have more than 5 inches of water in his or her bath at Buckingham Palace, and we patriotically followed the example given by the Royal Family. Friday night was both my bath night and hair-washing night. We used ordinary soap to wash our hair and there were no 'pampering' toiletries, 'smellies', conditioner or hair spray.

We needed warm clothing in the winter season, and most schoolchildren wore black, lined, gabardine raincoats made of good strong 'Utility' material, with the 'Utility' symbol of two three-quarter circles beside the number '41' printed on a label inside the garment. This signified the year 1941 when the 'Utility' clothes rationing system was brought into effect, limiting the amount of material used in a skirt or dress, and restricting the size of lapels on coats and suit jackets. It was intended to guarantee a certain quality and good value in the austerity item to which it was affixed, and the manufacturer only received permission by the Government to use this 'Utility' label if his goods were made to a satisfactory standard. Everyone had a clothes ration book containing sixty-six coupons that had to provide all the clothes for one person for a year.

I wonder what happened to our outgrown clothes? There were no charity shops to take them to. Outgrown clothes would be passed down to younger brothers or sisters, but I had no brothers or sisters and I don't remember having any of

Rose's outgrown clothes. I didn't know about Jumble Sales either - perhaps they were held at church halls. We didn't have Jumble Sales at our small, rented, part-time church.

Worn blouse or shirt collars were often unpicked, turned and carefully stitched back on again and worn for a little longer. A garment was only discarded, or the sound fabric used for some other purpose, when the material began to fray. Moths were a serious threat to woollen clothes and spare blankets were stored away in the summer months. The moths were busy laying their eggs in our cupboards and drawers, and the grubs grew fat by munching holes in our winter woollies. We used to chase any moths in the summer months whenever we saw them flying around indoors, and tried to squash them before they settled in our jumpers or blankets and laid their destructive eggs. Man-made fibres that strengthen fabrics and make ironing easier don't attract moths, but these had not yet been developed. One rarely sees a household moth nowadays. Like many of our garden birds, they have become an endangered species due to lack of suitable food - in this case, wool.

I had two grey school blouses at Junior School and two white ones when I moved on to my Senior School and one blouse for worn for an entire week. Men's business shirts had separate collars, and a clean collar could be attached each morning to the neckband of the shirt with a collar stud, removing the necessity of putting on a clean shirt each day. It greatly reduced the amount of washing that had to be done! My father wore the same shirt for a week. He used to roll up his shirtsleeves beneath the sleeves of the jacket of his navy-blue three-piece suit, so that the cuffs were not exposed to any dirt or dust when he leant across the counter at the shop. The restrictions and shortages, as well as the difficulties of washing and drying clothes, precluded the frequent changes of any clothing. Everyone had to 'make do and mend' and keep as clean as possible, but although we may have looked a bit drab, most people took care of their appearance and dressed as smartly and neatly as possible. Nobody had a wide range of clothes, unless they had contact with the 'spivs' and consequent access to the illegal 'black market'. Old pictures of the times, together with my recollections, indicate that people took the trouble to look well dressed. It was almost part of the war effort not to look shabby.

Girls wore woollen jumpers over their white blouses in the winter. These were sometimes hand-knitted at home, often in rather dull colours, as there was very little selection of either coloured wool or fancy knitting patterns. The arms of jumpers and cardigans were unravelled when they got a bit thin at the elbows or worn at the cuffs. The thin wool was discarded and the thicker wool was loosely wound into a skein, lightly washed to remove the wrinkles, and then rewound. The arms were re-knitted using the recycled wool, producing slightly shorter sleeves! Making-do with re-used wool was still a necessity long after the War had ended, and I can remember still doing this process when I hand-knitted my young sons' jumpers in the 1950s and early 60s.

'Auntie' didn't knit, but knitting was a popular pastime. I taught myself to knit, and my first effort was a 'pixy-hood' to wear to Junior School in the winter. Laboriously knitting a long scarf-like length on large needles and stitching up along one side for some inches from the middle eventually made a pointed head covering. Most of the girls in my School wore these 'pixy hoods' in severe weather. They protected our heads and ears, and when we tucked the ends into our coat collars they kept our necks warm too. They were not very becoming but keeping warm was much more important than being smart in cold weather. When I was a bit older I knitted several rather plain jumpers with the dull wool and simple patterns that were available. Girls sat by the fire during the evenings when their homework was finished, knitting while listening to the radio.

During the winter I wore thick, grey, woollen, calf-length socks to Junior School. They were turned over just below the knee and held up with elastic garters. They tended to slip down to the ankle and frequently had to be pulled up again. The saying, "Pull your socks up" had a literal meaning for the scruffy appearance of some small boys or girls. Older girls wore fawn, woollen or lisle, stockings that were also quite thick and secured with suspenders attached to a 'liberty' bodice. The liberty bodice had little to do with liberty but was another layer of clothing to insulate us from the cold. Why was it called a liberty bodice, I wonder? Stockings were inclined to stretch and soon wrinkled around the ankles, so these often needed pulling up too. Socks and stockings required frequent darning; there was always a pile of socks and stockings needing repair, and I did my own mending from quite a young age. I quite enjoyed this occupation, listening to the wireless while holding a wooden 'mushroom' over the hole with one hand and weaving the appropriate shade of fawn wool in and out with my needle with the other. I have almost forgotten that the task existed. Holes in heels and toes appeared frequently when people were on their feet so much in their daily tasks at home and at play, walking to work, to school and to the shops. Wool was not strengthened with a man-made fibre, and nylon had not yet appeared. Ladies wore unfashionable rayon stockings instead of the pre-war silk ones; ladders appeared easily and frequently and were a time-consuming occupation to repair - again and again.

Rose sometimes painted her legs with 'liquid stocking' when she was in her teens. Then she carefully drew a black line down the back of her legs to produce the illusion of a seam. Seams were no doubt thought to be 'sexy' (although nobody would have used this word!). They added to the attraction of good calves in the older girls, but straight seams were a sign of being 'properly dressed'. Even when we were still schoolgirls we always checked that the line on our stocking seams was straight before going out.

While her mother was working on Saturdays, Rose and I occasionally indulged in toast and butter for our tea, extravagantly spreading most of our weekly ration of butter on our toast. We sat close to the fire, holding our thick slices of bread on the end of the carving fork and a wire toasting rack close to the brightly glowing coals. Bread toasted very quickly in front of an open fire and seemed to have a much nicer taste than when done in a modern electric toaster today.

In spite of all the little deprivations in our daily lives we enjoyed occasional trips to the West End of London. Our winter visits to London were made after the Blitz was over and it was considered safe to travel to the capital again. Rail fares were relatively cheap and the train fare to London was unexceptional in wartime. (Even when I began working as a shorthand typist in 1947 and had a wage of £3 a week, I was given an additional travel allowance of 5s. [25p]. This almost covered the cost of my weekly season ticket to London).

'Auntie' had worked in one of the big stores as a bookkeeper in the past and 'Selfridges' and 'John Lewis' were her favourite stores. She loved the buzz of a trip to the West End - as did I. We especially enjoyed looking around the 'bargain basement' in Selfridges. The John Lewis store always seemed very old-fashioned to me, with several steps leading into the different departments, which made it difficult to find one's way around. I think it had developed little by little in earlier years, with the Company taking over adjacent shops and incorporating them into the large department store it eventually became. Both stores, along with a number of others in the West End, were bombed during the Blitz, and John Lewis's was totally rebuilt near Oxford Circus, but Selfridges still retains its original distinctive frontage.

Our journey to the West End took us on the Metropolitan Line from Northwick Park, our nearest station, to Baker Street Station. From there we walked down Baker Street and made for Selfridges in Oxford Street. In those days Selfridges was a good-value store for the ordinary customer. The Utility system prevented elaborate outfits or inflated prices in any shops and only British-made clothes were available. The customers were not necessarily wealthy and were certainly not foreign tourists! There were no luxury goods available. 'Auntie' was looking for new 'best' winter coats for both Rose and me on one trip to the West End. A lovely red all wool coat with cherry-shaped buttons down the front was bought for me and hidden away until Christmas, when I received it as my present from my father. I was very fond of this coat and wore it for 'Sunday best' for years. It was too long for me when it was new. The hem had to be turned up for the first season I wore it and was let down little by little as I grew taller. Children seemed to grow more slowly years ago and I don't remember ever having a replacement 'best' coat until I grew up.

Before we returned home from our day's outing to London we usually had a cup of tea in a Lyons teashop in Oxford Street. Occasionally we walked up to Lyons Corner House at Marble Arch, where 'Auntie' was able to rest her feet for a while and she, Rose and I enjoyed a cup of tea and perhaps a toasted teacake. A waitress, known as 'a nippy', in her little black dress and starched white frilly cap and apron, took our modest order as we sat at our table. While we waited for our pot of tea, we listened to 'live' music being played on a small raised stage by an elderly violinist and his accompanist, who were no doubt glad to be earning a little money in exchange for the entertainment they gave. It generated a light-hearted atmosphere that cheered us immensely before we began our journey home, walking up Baker Street again to the Underground station.

I noticed some bomb damage on our visits to London, with boarded up shops, some ruined property and empty spaces where buildings had been. I had none of the horror, however, that I experience today when I see pictures of terrorist activity in my own country, or any of the dismay and sorrow that I now feel when I see pictures of destruction elsewhere. As a child I seemed to be unaware of much of the terror and ghastliness of the War. Perhaps I just accepted the existing conditions of life as normal. Yet I was so conscious of the miseries of queuing and shopping, cold feet, chilblains and holes in socks!

When I came home from school I was very occasionally told that the greengrocer had received a delivery of oranges. Oranges never appeared during the summer months and the queue for oranges outside the greengrocer's on a cold winter's afternoon was always enormous. I often waited for an hour or two as I dreamed of the few oranges I hoped I would be taking home. Everyone in the queue was concerned that the fruit might all be sold before they were served. On one occasion Mr. Jackman's allocation of oranges ran out just as I had reached the outside of the shop window. It was such a let-down after all that queuing in the cold, rubbing my hands together and stamping my feet on the pavement to try and keep warm. The queue suddenly dispersed; everybody was bitterly disappointed, but also reasonably cheerful and accepting, but it was quite hard to have spent so long in the cold and then have to return home without the special treat that would have made it all worthwhile. At the time I had no idea of the dangers that the Merchant Fleet had suffered for these rare fruits to reach our shops.

I arrived home with freezing extremities, took off my coat, pixy hood and gloves and put my feet on to the opened front of the kitchen boiler. As I sat watching the flames dancing behind the grid, resting my cold feet on the top of the boiler, I could feel the heat gradually creeping through my shoes and warming my toes. This sometime resulted in scorch marks across the soles of my shoes and painful, red, swollen toes caused by the chilblains I suffered after this sudden change of temperature. The subsequent burning and itching in bed, when my feet grew really hot under the blankets and eiderdown became almost unbearable, and is unforgettable! I was glad of my hot water bottle on those wintry nights, but as it spent more time on my feet than the rest of my body. I am sure it aggravated my chilblains.

Children's shoes were not replaced as often as was necessary during the War and when I dressed in the mornings my swollen toes were sometimes squeezed into shoes that were a little too small. However, winter did not last forever, and when the spring came along our house had a pleasant sunny aspect. The big 'sun-trap' windows let in plenty of sunshine, light and warmth, and my recollections of wartime summers are of many long, hot, sunny days.

Chapter Twelve

CHRISTMAS MEMORIES

We made our home look bright at Christmas-time, and each December my father brought down from the loft a box of pre-war crepe paper Christmas decorations - bells and coloured paper lanterns. We made paper chains at Primary School, using brushes and jars of paste to stick the coloured strips together before joining them up to carry home excitedly at the end of term. We hung them from the corners of our living room to the centre light fitting. We bought holly from the greengrocers to drape over the top of the mirror above the fireplace and I can recall a bunch of mistletoe hanging in the hall - perhaps this was mainly for Rose's benefit when she became interested in boy friends! I have no remembrance of decorating a Christmas tree during my childhood either before, or during, the War.

My father opened the glass dividing doors between our two reception rooms on Christmas Day to promote a more party-like atmosphere, although we still only lit the one fire in the dining room to conserve fuel. One Christmas morning my father placed a small tray of drinks on the top of my mother's old sewing machine cabinet that was still tucked away behind the opened dividing glass doors. There was a bottle of sherry, a bottle of port and a bottle of Stone's ginger wine, with presumably some non-alcoholic drink for Rose and me. Perhaps Rose was becoming a slightly rebellious teenager, and when nobody else was around, she crept behind the folded glass doors, and began sampling the contents of one of the bottles. Her brief spell of secret drinking soon brought repercussions - she was found out and she became ill - or was it the other way round - she became ill before she was found out? This calamity brought a certain dampening of our spirits for a while, until Rose had recovered and been forgiven and the wine had been hidden away out of sight. A bottle of sherry lasted for a year or two in our house! Fruit juices, coke and squashes were not available; if we were thirsty, we usually had a glass of water.

English Cox's Orange Pippins were available during the late autumn and were a treat at Christmas time. 'Auntie' liked them polished until their skins gleamed and they were then displayed in a bowl on top of the gramophone cabinet - becoming almost a part of the Christmas decorations.

There were very few toys available during the War years, but we did give one another Christmas presents. My father usually gave me a new dress, maybe a pair of gloves or slippers, or some other garment I needed. The gifts I received were usually practical or useful, never frivolous or extravagant. My illustrated Authorised Version of the Bible was a Christmas present one year from 'Auntie'. I once received a Waterman's fountain pen and propelling pencil and proudly used these at Senior school instead of the nasty wooden school pens. I think my handwriting improved a little with this new pen and pencil. Rose gave me a copy of Dickens' 'Oliver Twist' one Christmas towards the end of the War, and she also gave me the music of Mendelssohn's 'Bees' Wedding' when my piano playing had advanced to that stage. I received a copy of 'Alice in Wonderland' in 1941 from Miss Skinner with whom I had lived when I was four years old. I still have it, inscribed inside, 'To Sheila from Miss Skinner, l94l'. I don't remember receiving this gift but I do have this evidence of her continued kindness and interest. The book is a wartime publication using inferior paper and with a few black and white illustrations, but it is the only book I remember receiving, and certainly the only one I still possess from my childhood years.

I can't recall any of the gifts I gave my father but I remember spending a long time trying to think what I could give him. I also spent a long time selecting 'Auntie's' present in our nearest Woolworth's, looking at their array of 'bath salts' displayed in large containers along the counter. They were only coloured and scented soda crystals but they seemed very exotic to me at the time. My mind wavered between the mauve, lavender-scented and the pink, rose-scented variety before I made my final decision. The pink was a very pretty colour but I knew 'Auntie' liked to use Yardley's Lavender

Water, so I settled on the lavender bath salts. They cost 4d. a pound, and were weighed up in scales by an assistant behind the counter before she poured them into a brown paper bag. I fear that my cheap perfumed soda crystals did not match the quality of her Yardley's products, but I can remember coming home very pleased with my purchase. I placed the crystals into a square collar box provided by my father before wrapping up my present. (Collars were stored in square cardboard boxes at the shop and discarded when empty. They made very useful gift boxes.) Did we have Christmas wrapping paper? I can't remember.

Christmas fare was limited. A chicken was likely to be a little 'elderly' and of uncertain tenderness, but scratching around in a farmyard for many months must have added taste if not tenderness to the flesh. We did have a roast chicken for some Christmas dinners and 'Auntie' was always concerned that it would be tender. She asked the butcher for a capon, which was a specially reared, castrated bird and was larger and more tender - the forerunner of battery-reared hens, perhaps? We never saw chicken thighs or breasts in the butcher's shop window, or ate a chicken casserole or chicken curry in those days. Chicken was a very special, rare, celebratory treat; it was always roasted and had real flavour that cannot be matched by the present day, rapidly produced poultry. Even organic or free-range poultry has little flavour compared with the chicken we used to have occasionally for our Christmas dinner. However, the mirror of my mind does not reflect any strong memory of what kind of meat was on our plates each Christmas - I only know it would not have been pork - but I can remember the pudding!

Our housekeeper always managed to find the ingredients for a Christmas pudding, and also a Christmas cake for tea. I used to sit at the side of the kitchen table watching her make this Christmas fare. We all joined in the traditional stirring of the pudding when we each made a wish. What did we wish for? - An end to the War?..... For my mother to get better? I think the latter wish was more of a formality than an expectation, as I don't think I had much hope of my wish being fulfilled. A few weeks later I watched intently as Auntie iced the Christmas cake.

The ingredients for these Christmas goodies were hoarded from some of our rations over the previous months. Sometimes a special allocation of dried fruit was given before Christmas. If we were able to obtain some muscatel raisins, they had to be carefully washed and the hard little stones removed from the large, succulent, dried fruit. This was one of my jobs, with the reward of an egg-cupful of raisins to eat afterwards. We occasionally had to use chopped prunes as a substitute for currants. The almond paste for the cake was made from soya flour, ground rice, sugar, dried egg and almond essence, and was a bit gritty and synthetic but the colour and texture were acceptable; nobody complained.

Christmas tea was a fairly simple meal. The 'best' tea service belonging to my parents was taken out of the china cabinet and placed on the table. The centrepiece was the iced and decorated Christmas cake placed on an elegant cake stand of 'Auntie's', and encircled with a colourful paper frill. It was not a very rich cake inside, but there was always sufficient fruit and darkness of colour from the addition of a little black treacle to make it look a luxury cake when it was cut, and it tasted good. 'Auntie' was proficient with her icing syringe and nozzles and always made an attractive seasonal design on the top of the cake.

A plate of bread and butter was prepared and put on the table - our measured portions being united for the occasion and the butter was spread on the bread in the kitchen. (When did I last see a plate of bread and butter? Afternoon tea has disappeared and been replaced with dinner, supper, snacks, or a take-away.) We had a glass vase in which were placed the stalks of a well-washed head of celery - an essential part of our wartime Christmas tea. We ate our bread and butter, and enjoyed the scrunch of the celery, with the added flavour from a little salt on the side of our tea plates into which we lightly dipped our stalk of celery. One could not buy many salad ingredients during the cold weather but celery was considered to be at its best after it had been blanched by a frost. It was covered with sooty dirt when we bought it from the greengrocer's. All the brown and blemished outside sticks were discarded and the remainder needed much scrubbing and cleaning before it was fit to eat. There was often very little of our head of celery left, but what we had was undoubtedly organic! (How different from the clean, uniformly sized, thick-stemmed, crisp celery heads we can buy all the year round nowadays.) We had a dish of homemade jam, or, if we had been in the Express Dairy at the right time, we might have some melon and ginger jam, which added a Christmassy, spicy flavour to our meal. We were occasionally lucky enough to have a small tin of salmon, if 'Auntie' had been able to use some of our precious 'points' in the grocer's shop when tinned salmon was in stock. If not we made do with a jar of 'salmon and shrimp', or 'sardine and tomato' fish-paste. I know that we would not have had any ham or Spam on our Christmas tea table!

We listened attentively to the King's speech on the radio after our Christmas dinner. A special 'Forces Favourites' was broadcast at noon on Christmas Day, relaying messages and music chosen by relatives of those serving in the Forces. We sometimes played Lexicon (a card game that was superseded by Kan-U-Go and then Scrabble some years after the War ended.) There was no television to watch in the evening, but, far, far better, was our own entertainment, when my father played some of his old waltz and fox-trot records on our wind-up gramophone and we danced around in the extra space our opened glass doors provided. I loved dancing the waltz and the foxtrot with my father. He had enjoyed ballroom dancing with my mother when they were younger, had taught me the correct steps for these old-fashioned dances, but sadly I didn't go to dances when I grew older.

We also played an improvised game of table tennis, propping up two or three collar-box lids across the centre of our extended dining-room table. An ashtray or some other small weighty object was positioned at each side of the cardboard to keep the lids upright. This formed a makeshift table tennis 'net', which enabled us to play a kind of table tennis. I don't know where my father procured the two bats and one or two balls from, or why we did not have a proper net, but I guess that new ones were unobtainable during the War. It was 'make do and play' as well as 'make do and mend'. It was only possible for two people to play at one time, as neither the table nor the room were wide enough for us to play doubles, but I really enjoyed this somewhat cramped and unorthodox form of table tennis after our Christmas tea. My father was a good player, with a very tricky left-handed serve. Despite the limitations of wartime and the absence of my mother, I look back on our Christmas festivities with much pleasure and we always seemed to have a very jolly time together.

A knock at the front door after the blackout curtains had been drawn was a rare occurrence at any time, but even more so at Christmastime. It was more than a little disconcerting to hear a loud bang, bang, bang, at our front door, interrupting our dancing late one Christmas evening. My father, rather hesitantly, went to the door and was greeted by a slightly tipsy Canadian soldier standing on our porch doorstep. This stranger explained that he had been walking down the road from the local public house after closing time and felt very homesick. He was missing his relatives in Canada, wanted to be part of a family and also wished to see the inside of an English home, and to know how the English spent Christmas. So he had wandered up our drive and knocked on our door. Perhaps he had heard our music or our laughter? After a little conversation, my father asked him in and explained to us why this unknown Canadian soldier was joining us. I think we were a little puzzled for a few moments by this unexpected guest, but our visitor seemed cheered by our welcome, pleased to have some company and to share in a little refreshment. After a while he left us and went on his way in the dark to his billet. I wonder what he thought of our low-key, homespun, improvised entertainment. I hope he had not been drawn to our house by a glimpse of light through our blackout curtains.

It was the custom for my father and me to visit my elderly Aunt and Uncle Connell at Mill Hill every Boxing Day. Wartime bus schedules and even more limited Christmas timetabling made for a very tedious journey by public transport, although the actual distance was only about ten miles. We stood at bus stops in freezing temperatures every Boxing Day morning. We had to change buses, often waiting a long time for our connection to Mill Hill and then had a long walk to my Uncle's house. It was an even colder and more miserable return journey in the evening, sitting in unheated, darkened buses as we travelled home. There was always a convivial Christmas atmosphere with these relations, and the same group of their friends was always present, but it was an all-adult house party. They were kindly people, but apart from me, my father was the youngest in the party. The house was decorated with dark green, glossy, holly boughs brought in from the garden and hung behind the pictures (also behind the dreaded antlers, which I still disliked although I had got over my earlier fear of them). My elderly Aunt and Uncle didn't have a Christmas tree and there were no colourful paper decorations either. We didn't sit in the lovely large drawing room that had seemed so elegant and comfortable before the War, but spent the day around the log fire in what had been known as the morning the room. We now also ate all our meals in this room, since the dining room had been transformed into my Uncle's office.

The usual procedure with the bottle of Graves wine occurred during the Boxing Day cold meal and the remains of the Christmas pudding still appeared, although not now doused in brandy and lit with gentle flame. There were still a few silver trinkets or silver threepenny pieces tucked inside the pudding and I always found some little silver treasure in my portion. After dinner the men played billiards in the cold drawing room as usual - and I got bored.

I never received a Christmas card from my mother, nor do I remember ever sending her one. Nobody suggested I should. No attempt was made to keep us in contact with each other. I didn't talk to anyone about her; she was not spoken about to me and I have no doubt that it was thought that we would never meet again. It must have been traumatic for her, incarcerated in the harsh environment of a psychiatric hospital at that period, and it seems possible that this lack of communication could have made her condition deteriorate still further. But maybe my birth was the cause of her illness and perhaps any contact would have been deemed unwise?

My father always visited her on the Sunday before Christmas, but apart from that he only saw her occasionally, as apparently her attitude towards him at that time was hostile and very aggressive. If seeing him made her more violent, then he felt it better to avoid visiting her too often. Perhaps it would have been better for him - and possibly for me - if he had divorced her and remarried? I am sure that he would not have considered this; his marriage vows were for faithfulness 'in sickness and in health until death us do part', but his loyalty was not appreciated. He was quite elderly before he told me that when he had driven home from work every lunch time when I was little, it was not only because I was not being cared for properly, but because my mother was suspicious of him and delusional. But I know that he was faithful to her throughout his life and always did what he felt to be the best for her welfare.

His Christmas visit to the Hospital was a wearisome, depressing experience, and I can recall him looking drawn and very tired when he came home. Waiting for public transport, sitting in the unheated bus, the stressful visit, followed by a return journey in the dark of a late December afternoon with very subdued, masked lighting in the buses, was no cheering lead up to his two-day Christmas holiday. He took her some little treats, a box of cakes, some sweets and a present of some new garment to wear, but I learned later that my mother often became violent at his appearance and refused to accept them. The packages had to be left with the Sister to give to her when she had calmed down after his departure. My father then returned to the hospital shortly after Christmas to make sure that she had been given his presents, that the clothes were suitable, and that she was able to wear the dress or cardigan, or whatever it was he had brought for her.

These visits always required an early Sunday dinner for us all, so that my father could catch his bus and train connections and reach the Hospital for the fixed visiting hours between 2 and 3.30 p.m. Sometimes he made the long journey, had an unpleasant reception, handed over his parcels to the Sister and left almost immediately. I had no real knowledge at the time of how my mother was behaving, but I can still sense the tension and his anxiety before, and more especially, after, those Sunday visits, and gleaned some idea of his reception from snippets of conversation I overheard with our housekeeper. The only communication I was involved in on these occasions was when I asked my father before he left home to, "Give Mumma my love". I never thought to send her a note or a real message.

On his return I usually asked him, "How was Mumma today?". His reply never changed, "About the same dear". There was little else he could say. He never brought back a message from my mother to me. He had seen his wife in a locked Ward, which would have been full of equally, or perhaps even more severely, ill ladies, who were unfortunate enough to suffer from some form of serious psychiatric illness. What was their Christmas like? Were they given some special treats? Would they be able to appreciate any pleasant change in their Ward routine? Was Christmas Day any different from any other day in the restricted environment of the hospital, with locked Wards and sometimes-violent patients? Would my mother have thought about previous Christmases when she was at home and well? How many of the ladies in my mother's Ward would even have received visits from their relatives? They were largely a forgotten community. This pre-Christmas visit was not a very auspicious start to our celebrations, but my father seemed able to put it behind him once Christmas Day arrived and we did have happy times at Christmas.

My few relations usually sent me Postal Orders for Christmas and my first duty after the festivities was to write my 'thank you' letters. I composed each letter carefully and was expected to write something appropriate and interesting as well as expressing a mere 'thank you'. I sat at the dining table, penning my little epistles in my best handwriting (especially to my teacher uncle in Devonshire). Writing letters of thanks was a task that most children were expected to complete, but it hung over our heads as a cloud in the school holidays until every one had been written, the envelopes addressed and the letters had been sent off to their various destinations. The rest of our holiday was our own - apart from the 'helping' tasks around the home that were expected of most children.

Chapter Thirteen

JUNIOR SCHOOL DAYS

In 1938 I had moved from the Infants' into the junior section of Priestmead Junior Mixed and Infants' School. There were two completely independent Priestmead Schools at the time, each with its own Headmistress, both sharing the same site and the same name. The more modern school was a brick building, constructed when the area was being developed in the early nineteen-thirties. I never met the Headmistress of this school but she was reputedly a very formidable lady and an active member of the Communist Party. She stood unsuccessfully as a candidate for Parliament in the General Election soon after the end of the War. Although I had no idea of what a Communist meant or what the Party stood for I can recall the *frisson* of shock in the neighbourhood when we heard that Miss Driver was standing for Parliament.

I attended the 'other' Priestmead School, which comprised a number of wooden, prefabricated structures and was always referred to as 'The Huts'. These supposedly temporary classrooms were erected when houses were first built in what had been a rural area, but even these two schools were found to be inadequate after the rapid development of housing in the early thirties. Before I started School in 1936 a number of children, including the boy who became my husband many years later, were taught in the local cricket pavilion for some of their Primary School years.

'The Huts' seem to me now to be more like an old TB sanatorium than a school but they were probably old First World War army huts. The long rows of black-treated wooden classrooms had open-fronted timber verandas providing plenty of fresh air as we moved around the school corridors. The Infant Department had similar covered but open-sided timber terraces in front of their classrooms, giving wet weather protection to everyone as they moved about the single-storey buildings. Additional covered verandas in the

Infant School bridged across two long blocks of classrooms, leaving small square spaces in between for groups of young children to play in safety. I had spent my first two years of education in this protective and yet open environment.

It was quite unlike any school I have seen since, but at the time it was the only kind of school I knew. After I had entered the Junior School, I sometimes looked across the playground with envy towards the large, modern, brick building that was quite alien to the experience of those of us in 'The Huts'. I didn't quite understand why there was this great 'divide' between the two Schools. We soon learned of the fierce reputation of Miss Driver in 'The Bricks', but I much preferred the gentler approach of our own headmistress, Miss Daly, who led our morning Assemblies with prayers and a hymn each day. The sound of our youthful voices singing, "Morning has broken, like the first morning" must have wafted across to the nearby homes on many occasions. Miss Daly was a far more approachable lady, and I sometimes saw her walking along Kenton Lane to the bus stop after school. This made her seem quite 'human' and 'normal' and I dared to say "Good afternoon, Miss Daly" if I met her in the street.

The road I lived in was the dividing line for two catchment areas. Those on one side of Kenton Lane, together with the children living in the adjacent streets to the West, went to the 'The Bricks'. Those living on the opposite side of the road and in the streets to the East were nearer to 'The Huts'. Many children in the more superior building of the 'Bricks' were not even aware that the modest huts at the lower end of their playground was a School! I was allocated to this prefabricated school building. There was no parental choice. My church was 'The Hut' and my school was 'The Huts'! Amazingly, the 'temporary' wooden classrooms of my Infant and Junior School were still being used when my own sons began their Primary education at the same School in the 1960s, when there was still no parental choice of Primary School. By this time however, 'Huts' and 'Bricks' had amalgamated into one school, with one Head Teacher, and pupils spent only a small part of their Primary years in the hutted classrooms. At last the envy that the children in the 'Huts' had for their better-housed fellow pupils had disappeared, and the divisive element that had existed between the two Schools in my day was eliminated. On visiting the area and looking at where my old school had been, it is difficult to imagine that the black timber classrooms had ever existed. A much larger playground has swallowed up my old hutted School. All that remains is a long strip of grass, which was our School garden during the War. This was where we helped to 'dig for victory', but it is now very difficult to visualise our gardening sessions.

The School colours were identical for pupils of the 'Huts' and the 'Bricks', and all pupils in the Junior School wore a grey and red striped tie together with a grey shirt or blouse, and grey and red stripes around the tops of our grey knee-length woollen socks. All the boys wore short, grey worsted trousers throughout their Primary School years and the girls wore black gymslips with three box pleats at the front and the back. Boys always wore a cap with the School badge on and girls wore a black velour hat, adorned with the School badge during the winter and some wore a Panama hat in the warm summer weather. Boys' clothing remained the same throughout the year. School uniform was worn by most children, but was not compulsory and cotton dresses were the usual attire for the girls during warm weather.

Rose and I were never allowed to begin wearing summer dresses, or to leave our vests off, until 'May was out'. Rose and I had many arguments about the meaning of the word 'May' – it meant the 'May' blossom (very likely), or the First of May (possibly), but certainly not the end of the month of May. I think that Rose, being older, quietly disobeyed her mother, but I always felt I should obey the rules! Consequently I sometimes sweltered in a wool vest on a warm day!

Crates of milk were delivered to the school by Brazier's Farm early every morning and placed outside each classroom door. At 'playtime' some of the bigger boys dragged a large metal crate of milk from the veranda to the front of the classroom. Each child received one third of a pint of milk free of charge, and when the 'playtime' bell was rung we each collected our bottle of milk and a straw. We pressed a little hole through the middle of the round cardboard disc at the top of the bottle and then pushed the straw into the milk. In the winter, the crates of bottles were dragged into the classrooms before the register was called, and pulled close to the stove in order to take the chill off the milk before our mid-morning break, as it was icy cold and sometimes partially frozen. But it was still very cold when we drank it! On very hot summer days there was a thick layer of creamy milk at the top of the bottle and we would have relished a chunk of frozen milk to chill the tepid morning drink, but I am sure we all benefited from the nutrition it provided.

The old classrooms in 'The Huts' were very difficult to heat adequately in the winter because of their structure and the open corridors of the school. The children sat in long rows of double desks in the Junior School classrooms, and a small hole in the right-hand corner of each pupil's desk contained a ceramic inkwell. A monitor was responsible for keeping each inkwell filled. There was no proper central heating, and warmth was not easily generated or sustained in such an open situation. An old, black stove in each classroom was supposed to heat the whole room and pipe heat to some radiators, but was very inefficient. During the War the School occasionally ran out of fuel for these old stoves. As soon as we entered our classroom on cold, frosty mornings, we would rush to our desks and push our penholders into the inkwells, hoping to discover that the ink had frozen. If this had occurred, we were all sent home for the day, as it was considered to be too cold for us to work in such low temperatures. By today's standards it seems rather a crude way of checking the temperature! We had the luxury of a day free from lessons but we were unlikely to be much warmer at home. We also needed every available hour of education to make up for our enforced loss of schooling at the beginning of the War and during the Blitz.

Each pupil was provided with a wooden penholder into which was pushed a metal nib. If I pressed too hard on to my exercise book as I wrote, the nib soon crossed at the tip and produced scratchy handwriting. It was even more easily damaged if it was poked too forcefully into the inkwell, or if the ink was powdery and lumpy. We had to write with the nib until it was almost impossible to use any longer, and new nibs were given out reluctantly. Each pupil also had a small square of blotting paper which had to last until it was saturated with inkblots, or crumpled through being pressed on to our writing or arithmetic books too frequently. Our teacher examined our work before a new piece was given, but neat work, good handwriting and figures were still expected of us.

Every time I needed to dip my pen into the inkwell I had to reach across to the right side of my desk because I was left-handed and consequently often made blots over my work. I had an unsteady left hand and found it difficult to write neatly. My father had developed 'writer's cramp' through having to write out the hand-written bills for customers at the shop very rapidly, and so he had to learn to use his left hand. He developed a very distinctive, but wobbly, backward-slanting handwriting, but detested writing letters as he found fine hand control difficult. I know the problem! I can only remember my father writing with his left hand, but often wonder whether he, too, was by nature left-handed, and whether his 'writer's cramp' was caused through being made to use his right hand when he was a child.

I was having difficulty in mastering 'joined-up writing' in my first year of Junior School and one day my class teacher made some very uncomplimentary remarks about my handwriting in front of the whole class. I explained to him that I was left-handed, hoping that this would excuse my bad writing. He suggested that I used my other hand, and said he would remember to make some allowances about the quality of my written work as I practised with my right hand. I adored this fair-haired, handsome young teacher, Mr. Flowers, who was the only male teacher in the school. I agreed to try, but after my initial attempt to make my right hand move in a controlled way, my next piece of work was a real mess. When our English books were handed out, this much-admired teacher was very scathing about my terrible handwriting. He had forgotten our agreement to make some concessions during my initial attempts to use my right hand. My exercise book was covered in red-inked comments about my careless writing. I was heart-broken that he had not kept his word, and had been so displeased with my efforts. I felt I would never forgive him - until he was called up into the Forces the following year and disappeared from school. He came back to see us on one occasion looking very smart in his RAF uniform, but we never saw him again. I hope that he survived the War.

I still have my school report for the year ending July 1939 informing me that my position was ninth in a class of forty-one children when Mr. Flowers was my class teacher. This was the year my mother had once again been admitted to hospital, so I had not done too badly considering the strains and stresses that there must have been at home in the preceding months. I wonder whether Mr. Flowers knew about my home circumstances. My report also states that I was absent from school only once during the year and late four times. What was the reason for my late arrival, I wonder? It may have been through problems at home, or after my mother had gone back into hospital, when my father had to 'deliver' me to a neighbour before going to work himself. My teacher's comment on my report was that 'Sheila would do even better if she made up her mind to work hard all the time'. As I received the comments 'Good' or 'Very good' for six of the nine subjects listed in my report I think he might have been a little more encouraging! My early delight in learning poetry seems evident in my grading of 'Very Good' for Recitation. There was far more information on this report than on my later Wartime Junior School reports. The two subsequent Priestmead School Reports were only half the size of the one I received in 1939 and were sparse in detail.

Miss Darlow was my class teacher in my Second Year (Year 4), whom I also liked very much, and my interest in poetry grew in her class. Several of the poems I read or learned then still come to mind and give me pleasure from time to time. 'The Listeners' by Walter de la Mare, 'Cargoes' by John Masefield were great favourites, particularly some of the lines in the latter poem, as I visualised the 'Stately Spanish galleon, coming from the Isthmus, Dipping through the tropics by the palm green shores'. I did not realise the significance of the 'firewood' mentioned in the third verse when I recited, 'Dirty British coaster, with a salt-caked smoke stack; Butting through the Channel in the mad March days, With a cargo of Tyne coal, road-rail, pig lead, Firewood, ironware and cheap tin trays'. I didn't know then that firewood had been the business of my unknown grandfather. I just enjoyed the sound of the words, the rhythm of the lines and the pictures the poem painted in my imagination.

I also loved, but never understood, a poem called 'Overheard on a Saltmarsh' by Harold Munro that we learned in another class. It had a mystery about it and the poem haunted me over many years, although I could only remember tiny snatches of it, little phrases such as 'Green glass, goblin', 'Give them me, give them...No!' I never came across this poem again until I saw it quite recently in a little anthology of Childhood Poems. I bought the book especially to enjoy the pleasure of reading this one particular poem, which I had not read since I was eight or nine years old. So many of the poems we learned at school are stored in the back of my mind and fragments can still be recalled. It may be disapproved of now, and may have seemed tedious at the time, but memorised poetry has provided many of my generation with much delight throughout our lifetime.

Miss Darlow was particularly interested in our progress in English and I began to appreciate all aspects of these lessons when in her class and even enjoyed the formal grammatical exercises we used to do. Creative writing was called 'composition' when I was at school and I once had to write about 'The Life Story of a Penny' - a penny would go a long way and could have quite an adventurous life in a young schoolgirl's imagination then. Our teacher had a very pleasant, lilting voice, and we had elocution lessons from time to time to improve our diction. Everyone had to bring a small mirror to school, and we sat at our desks with our mirrors in front of us, intently watching the shape of our mouths as we repeated individual vowel sounds, or recited some alliterative rhymes - 'The rain in Spain falls mainly on the plain', or 'How now brown cow'. We looked at the shape of our lips as we said, 'ai' and 'ow', while concentrating on sounding the ends of words clearly. Perhaps the present generation would benefit from such simple exercises as these? I find a distinct lack of clarity in speech nowadays and the speed often makes it quite unintelligible.

We learned our tables of number meticulously and regularly recited them in unison in our arithmetic lessons. We were given ten mental arithmetic questions to do immediately after Assembly every morning and these exercised our brains, as we wrote our answers down very quickly. I think we all dreaded the daily 'dose', but nearly burst with pride if we were able to tick our correct (or mainly correct) answers. I am sure that I was not the only one who found some of my Primary School arithmetic rather difficult to grasp, (as my grade in Mr. Flowers' class appeared to confirm). 'Problems' were particularly tricky. Trying to work out how many gallons of water would be needed to fill a bath in a certain time seemed rather pointless to young children – especially when we couldn't have a bath full of water!

I found long multiplication sums easy, probably because I knew my tables well and the rows of figures formed a neat column as the calculation progressed. When it came to learning long division, I was good at the initial estimation required, which saved a lot of time in completing the sum correctly and I liked the long 'tail' of figures that developed as I worked out the sum. I have subsequently always been much better at having, hopefully, inspired but reasonably accurate estimations in real life mathematical situations. Fractions appeared easy to me and again knowing my 'times' tables was a great help, but I was taught nothing about metrication. A lot of emphasis was put on knowing the four rules of number – addition, subtraction, division and multiplication - together with our tables of number, weight, measurement, length and time. Some of these tables were rather complicated and had many different terms and irregularities, which made them difficult to memorise. Rods, poles or perches were never required in my daily experience and I didn't have much to do with furlongs, bushels or hundredweights either (although I knew that our coal was delivered in one hundredweight sacks). How much simpler is the metric system - but how much easier it is for those who grew up with Imperial weights and measures to understand and use pounds and ounces, pints and quarts, yards, feet and inches. They are more tangible and natural measurements to most of my generation than milligrams, litres, metres and kilos!

We had no calculators in our classrooms, only an ink-stained wooden ruler, although a cardboard 'tables' square' was allowed in the lower Junior School classes. Arithmetic at Primary School never progressed to any other branch of mathematics and there was little opportunity for practical work. We had our noses in our 'sum' books, our pens grasped in our hands and our minds were on our 'problems'. Our simple forays into algebra or geometry were not understood as such by us at the time, and our Arithmetic lessons were never called Maths.

Little comes back to my mind about the content of our Geography lessons, apart from a mental picture of an old school atlas showing a map of the world. Much of it was deep pink in colour - that was the British Empire. We collected labels from tins of food that showed their country of origin and I was delighted to be able to add a label from a tin of dark purple plums from Oporto in Portugal to the display table in the classroom. The War put an end to imported fruit from Europe and I very much doubt that I had any idea where Portugal was at the time. It must have been the closest we came in our day to doing any form of topic work, but it is interesting that the one fact I clearly remember about Junior School Geography is that Portugal exported purple plums from Oporto – even if I didn't know where it was! I have no other specific recollections of what we learned about our own land or any other countries.

We were taught about Stone Age Man, the Saxons and the Romans in our History lessons. I don't know whether all the facts I have retained in my mind are from my own schooldays, from my two sons' Junior School books, or reinforcements from the history textbooks used by the children I taught in Junior School myself some thirty years later. A lot of information is absorbed and becomes part of one's general knowledge, without recognising its source. I know that I enjoyed History much more when I taught it, and enjoy and understand it even more from reading historical novels.

We learned how to do cross-stitch, blanket stitch and chain stitch in our Needlework lessons, using brightly coloured threads and squares of cream, coarsely woven material called Binca. At first we made little mats, then larger tray cloths in the same material. We also made small articles such as egg cosies and pencil cases in brightly coloured felt, practicing our newly-learned simple embroidery skills. I preferred this form of needlework to the hems and seams, and attempts at garment-making that were to come in my secondary education. Perhaps similar little articles are still sewn nowadays in Primary School and proudly brought home at the end of term, but by boys as well as girls. Boys did not do needlework in my days at school - it was '*girls*' work - but I have no idea what craftwork the boys went off to while we had our more intimate, all-female sewing lessons. I have no memory at all of any Art lessons.

I thoroughly enjoyed my Music lessons, particularly the singing. I was less enthusiastic about the classroom instruments that were brought out from time to time and handed out for our use. The drums were usually given to the boys and tambourines were rather scarce. I seem to remember there were many more triangles, and I rarely seemed to get anything interesting to play. The sound we made was not very inspiring or tuneful - and probably not even very rhythmical! We sang a variety of songs in our Singing lessons, ranging from English folk songs, to 'Where the bee sucks, there suck I; In a cowslip's bell I lie'. I was quite oblivious at the time as to the identity of the illustrious poet who wrote the words of this song. We sang a number of songs from our National Song Book, including, 'It was a Lover and His Lass', 'Polly Oliver', the 'Miller of Dee' and sea shanties like 'Shenandoah' and 'Bobby Shafto'. We didn't learn about the background of these songs, or understood their meaning, but just appreciated the melody. We didn't snigger or giggle at the sentiments expressed in some of the songs. We knew nothing about jilted lovers, romance, or love affairs when we sang 'Early One Morning, just as the sun was rising', which was a favourite folk song of mine and is still remembered and enjoyed. We knew nothing about sex in Junior School, and I certainly didn't bother to try to understand why the poor abandoned maid down in the valley was sighing, 'Oh don't deceive me, oh never leave me; how could you treat a poor maiden so.'

We had an alternative version of the words of 'The Ash Grove', which is probably not unique to my old school. As we walked home after lessons were over, we often sang uproariously, 'My teacher's got a bunion, a face like a pickled onion; a nose like a squashed tomato, and legs like two sticks', to the tune of 'The Ash Grove'. This version was certainly not the love song of a jilted lover! We were obedient and dutiful in class but we did let off steam when away from the eyes and ears of our teachers, and often sang school songs or popular music heard on the radio as we tramped home after school to our tea. I can't remember the last time I heard children singing in the street.

Some music is timeless. It was just as satisfying to sing the familiar words of 'It was a Lover and his Lass', in a two-part setting by Imogen Holst with the fifty++-aged ladies Senior Singers' choir I belonged to for many years, as when I was in my class of forty plus ten-year-olds so many years ago. Music is no respecter of age and gives pleasure to old and young, but I do wonder how much of today's music will still be remembered or sung in over fifty years' time, and whether today's children learn many of our old traditional national songs.

It is interesting to consider the life-long effects that can ensue from some of the, seemingly, minor parts of one's early experience and education. I have gained pleasure from poetry throughout my life; this interest was certainly nurtured in school but I realise that I often listened to my father reciting some of the poems he remembered from his school - or night school - days. My delight in reading grew out of the hours I spent surrounded by books in the hushed surroundings of the local Library, as well as the books I borrowed to read at home. My love of music and singing was influenced not only by our school lessons, but also through hearing my father giving voice to all the old songs he loved and through listening to his old 78rpm classical records. I heard Tchaikovsky's 1812 Overture on the radio recently and my mind went back to the times when my father wound up his old gramophone before carefully placing the needle on the record.

Another lesson was introduced into the curriculum as the War proceeded. Gardening suddenly appeared on our timetable, although it was not indicated on our School Report. We had no test on our prowess in the school garden, or mark or grade to indicate the success of our exertions. We were encouraged to grow vegetables for the War effort, and I enjoyed these periods out in the sunshine, when we were 'doing our bit' and 'digging for victory'. There was the opportunity to chat whilst bending over our forks and hoes, but one day my teacher caught me talking to Bobbie Keogh. We both had to plunge our forks into the ground, leave our work and stand facing the black wooden school buildings. This was no real hardship, although we were supposedly in disgrace and separated from our hard-working classmates. It was very pleasant to stand in the sun and peep occasionally at everyone weeding, digging and hoeing, whilst having further little whispered conversations with each other when our teacher wasn't looking. We thought our punishment was very slight as we watched the rest of the class with their heads down, bent on their manual labour, although I may have felt a slight degree of disgrace, which is long forgotten, at being segregated from the rest of my classmates.

The playground was an exciting place but it could be a little dangerous during icy weather or after snow had fallen. It sloped gently over a large area between 'The Bricks' and down towards the 'Huts'. When there had been a snowfall or a very heavy frost, the boys slid down this long slope until its surface became like glass. Adventurous boys spent their entire playtimes whizzing along this slide. There were plenty of grazed knees but I don't remember any serious accidents. Another glassy slide was made by repeatedly sliding along another patch of ice; this second one was not quite as long and had only a barely noticeable gradient. It was therefore much less dangerous and some of the girls joined the more timid boys in sampling the thrills of this easier - 'B Grade' - slope. I suppose there was someone on duty, but I don't remember much intervention in our activities until a teacher appeared with a large handbell, ringing it vigorously to indicate the end of our playtime, when we hurriedly formed up into long class lines. There were no Health and Safely Regulations in force and no compensation culture if accidents occurred. At other seasons during the year we played the usual children's games with our balls, skipping ropes, cat's cradle, conkers, or chased around energetically playing 'he'.

Our annual School Reports for 1940 and 1942 were printed on very small pieces of paper, each measuring only l0cm x l4cm. We had no Report at all in l94l, the year of the Blitz. Primary School education came to an end in the summer of l942. My last Junior School report gives no marks at all for any tests, only comments of Very Good, Good or Fairly Good, for Progress, Attendance, Conduct, plus English Oral, English Written, Reading, Arithmetic and Handicraft. The number of pupils in the class is omitted, no individual position in class is indicated, and absences and lateness are not shown, as in the 1939 Report. I presume that this insignificant report was due to shortage of paper. Paper of all kinds was very scarce. Paper for exercise books was of inferior quality and I guess that there was little available for school reports. We must also have been far behind in our basic subjects because of the time lost in the classroom due to the War. Our core curriculum was very much 'core' and little else!

My final Report records that my progress was considered 'Very Good' and my conduct 'Good'. (Perhaps I had lost the 'very' because of talking in gardening class!) My teacher, Mrs. O'Callaghan's comment on this small scrap of paper was brief. It stated that 'Sheila has worked well this year. She has taken pride in her books and has made good progress'. There is no remark by my Headmistress, only Miss Daly's signature. When I consider all the upheavals in my first eleven years I feel that my father must have been quite pleased to receive this report despite its brevity. I have no idea whether my Headmistress or my teachers were aware of my mother's illness or my home circumstances over the years. I am not aware that anyone at school knew that my mother was in a Mental Hospital, but I remember feeling embarrassed, inwardly hurt and upset at school when classmates made thoughtless or sarcastic remarks about 'loony bins' or 'mad-houses' but I don't think this was personal taunting, I still find it distressing and so insensitive when adults make disparaging remarks about the mentally ill. People should now know better.

I have happy memories of my primary school years and liked and respected all my teachers. In spite of the limitations and restrictions that the War had imposed on our education and the distress and loss in my own life, I was not conscious of the former and had adjusted to the latter. I now rarely thought of my mother and I don't think I consciously missed her at all. She had almost been erased from my memory.

County Schools had many fee-paying parents and the only chance of free entry to a 'County' School was through passing the 'Scholarship' Examination, until the 1944 Education Act introduced equal educational opportunities for all. Not every child at Junior School was able to sit this Examination, and only a few children passed, but I was hoping – half expecting - to go on to the local County School. Because of the good

standard of my work I had not been required to
called the 'Preliminary' exam, which eliminated
were unlikely to pass the main Examination.
in the necessary forms and had chosen Harrow ᴄᴏ
School. There were few County Schools in the area ᴛ
choose from at this period, and I was aware of only the one traditional single sex School. The alternative co-educational County School was at Harrow Weald and was rather a difficult journey from home; my father had considered the other County Schools in Kingsbury and Pinner to be too far away. Neither parents nor prospective pupils were given the opportunity of a prior visit to any Senior or Secondary School in order to make an informed choice.

On a wet Saturday morning in February 1942, my friend Joan and I set off by bus to sit the main Entrance Examination at Harrow County School. We had been given instructions on how to find our way to the School and were a little anxious as we travelled on the 140 bus from Kenton Library to Harrow. We alighted at the right stop and had been told to turn right at the top of the town, so we walked up the main street towards the far end of the town. The Railway Bridge was as far as we had previously been and we assumed that this was the top of the town shopping centre, so we turned right immediately after the Bridge into what we thought was the road leading to the School. We soon realised that we were walking along a narrow service road beside the railway line that didn't appear to lead anywhere, and certainly didn't take us to Harrow County Girls' School.

We hastily retraced our steps, walked into unknown territory right up to the top of the main street, found the correct turning on our right - Sheepcote Road - and so reached the rather imposing entrance to the Harrow County Girls' School. We were not late - but not early either - and the cloakroom was already crammed full of seemingly identical damp, navy blue gabardine raincoats and black velour hats. We hung up our outdoor clothes on top of some others and were led into the Examination Hall, where most of the candidates were already seated. The room was hushed, and I felt a little daunted as I as shown to my desk. I glanced around the hall at all the other girls who were sitting there quietly, looking equally nervous and waiting for the examination to start. The examination Papers were handed out and we were told that there should be no talking and that we could begin. I turned my Paper over and studied it. I worked my way through the various questions and thought I had tackled everything reasonably well. I had no inkling that I had not acquitted myself favourably. After the examination had finished Joan and I, and others from my school, chatted on the bus home about the tests we had just done. I had very little doubt that I would be going to the County School the following September.

Some weeks later I came into our kitchen at breakfast time and my father told me that the postman had been and pointed to an envelope propped up against the little old clock on the window ledge. My expectations were completely shattered when I took the letter out of the buff envelope and read the contents. I had *failed* the examination to go to County School and was to attend Chandos Senior Girls' School instead. I could not believe it, but I hid my dismay, pretended I didn't mind, and went off to school with a smiling face.

Soon after I arrived at school my Headmistress called me to her office - a very unusual occurrence. I had never spoken to Miss Daly in school before and had only greeted her politely when I occasionally saw her as she walked along the road past my home. I stood quaking at the knees as I waited outside her office, wondering what I had done wrong, but when she called me inside she just asked me gently if I had been feeling unwell on the day of the examination. I could think of no reason to excuse my failure. Perhaps our brief loss of direction on our way to the School may have upset my concentration, but I was not unduly concerned at the time and didn't like to tell my Headmistress of our little mishap. Miss Daly told me how surprised she was that I had failed the Examination and suggested that my father queried the result. She spoke to me again at the end of term and when she heard that my father had made no enquiry, she urged me to take the 'over-age' examination the following year. This gave a second chance to pupils who may have been late-starters, or mis-placed originally. I assured her that I would do this.

Some time later it was rumoured that after our examination papers had been scrutinised, preference was given to children whose fathers were in the Forces. I have no knowledge as to whether there was any truth in the rumour, but I am inclined to believe that some kind of blunder might have occurred. I do remember that two girls who were never near the top of my class, and whose fathers were in the Forces, did go to Harrow County School, but perhaps their parents were able to pay the School fees. A few years later many new Grammar Schools had been built, the 11+ examination was introduced and everyone with the ability to benefit from an academic secondary Education had an equal chance of receiving it. What a difference a few years made to the opportunity of a good education!

At the time the alternative Senior Schools provided a less academic curriculum and were considered by many people to give an inferior education. A certain stigma was said to be experienced by parents whose children did not pass the 'Scholarship' examination for entry to a County School; they felt their children were failures and their offspring sometimes thought they were too. I was not aware of this at that time, and don't think that my father felt this, but in later years I have greatly regretted my lack of a Grammar School education and have felt diminished for most of my adult life because of it.

Before the implementation of the 1944 Education Act young people left their Senior School at fourteen years of age with little opportunity of any higher education, other than taking on an apprenticeship, doing a course at a Technical or Commercial College, entering the Civil Service or a Bank at the lower levels, with opportunities for advancement through courses and internal exams. There was a very limited selection of evening classes available. This Act was prepared during the dark days of the War and it was gradually implemented from 1945 onwards.

Deep inside I was very disappointed and ashamed of myself for failing the 'Scholarship' examination, but I believe that my father was not unduly upset. He may have been relieved that he would not have to find the money for the obligatory extras and expensive uniform that would be required at Harrow County School. The additional years of education that this School demanded would have put further strain on his finances. He may possibly have feared that an academic education, with its demands for more study and homework, would put too much stress on me in view of my mother's illness and my somewhat unsettled life. I think that would have been an incorrect assumption, as I have always enjoyed study and learning new things. There was no discussion or commiseration at home about my failure to pass the Scholarship Examination, and my father did not follow up my Headmistress's suggestion to query my results. The general public was somewhat in awe of 'authority' in those days. Maybe he, too, hid his disappointment, but I don't think he considered a good education was necessary for girls. Although most women were working during the War, he knew that most girls left work when they married a few years after leaving school. I am sure he had no idea of the depth of my dismay.

The opportunity of a challenging career was uncommon even for the majority of girls who received a Grammar School education; and it was almost unheard of in our experience for anyone to go to University. (I knew of nobody who went to University until after I was married, when our next-door neighbour's son went to Nottingham University early in the 1950s. My father thought it very strange that Alan did not leave school and go to work to bring in some extra money to help his parents bring up his two younger sisters!) Neither future ambition, nor a fulfilling career had entered my head at the time; I just wanted to go to what I thought would be a 'good' School.

Thus another period in my life ended. My Junior School days were over and the long summer holidays began. They seemed so long in those days and children helped around the house and generally amused themselves. After the holidays I would start on a new pathway in my life. Thoughts of education faded as I enjoyed myself in my recreational activities.

Chapter Fourteen

YOUTHFUL PURSUITS

I spent many hours of my spare time in our local recreation ground playing on the swings, the slide, the seesaw, the roundabout and the American swing. I loved pushing my legs higher and higher into the air on the swings and feeling the slight sinking feeling in my stomach when I propelled myself a bit too high. The long, shiny metal slide was very popular too. After waiting patiently on the iron steps, slowly reaching the top, a very quick decision had to be made to sit down at the edge of the slide and set off down the slippery slope. Others behind were impatient to have their turn and there was no time for hesitation. Bigger boys sometimes tried to take control of the American swing, pushing it to its full extent as the girls sitting along the bench screamed with excitement, mixed with a little fear. I sat on the roundabout, chatting or joking with friends as we gripped the metal bars to push it around or jerk it in and out. I usually arrived home with a distinct metallic smell on my grubby hands from grasping various pieces of the iron equipment.

Jock, the ever-vigilant park attendant, kept his eye on everyone and we often saw him waving his stick at the first sign of bullying or any misbehaviour. He made the bigger boys get off the swings if they attempted a male take-over or pushed them dangerously high, but he failed to notice a group of naughty little girls one afternoon when I tore the back of my dress scrambling over a bit of rough fencing. We were playing hide-and-seek and I thought I had found a good hiding place. Jock's watchful eye was on the older boys and he had not noticed me clambering about behind the big wooden shelter, where on rainy days we sat chatting under cover on the long wooden bench. I caught the back of my dress in a piece of jagged wood at the back, and had to go home with a huge tear right across the skirt of my summer dress – with the added embarrassment of revealing my navy blue knickers. After the dress had been mended I had to wear it to school for the rest of the week, while my second cotton dress was being washed and ironed. The tear was so large that the repair was rather obvious, and I felt very embarrassed when wearing the dress every other week for the rest of the summer. 'Auntie' had made two cotton summer dresses for me to wear for school, and I can still remember the pattern of my favourite one – the torn one - but there were no spare clothing coupons to buy material for a replacement for the torn dress.

Jock had not noticed my little escapade as he stood outside his little hut leaning on his stick, keeping an eye on - nearly - everyone. We were all a little bit frightened of him but he kept a crowd of youngsters in order very effectively. None of us owned a watch and we would ask him to remind us of the time when we were expected to leave the park and go home for our tea. He seemed to remember to call out, "Time to go home", and point his stick at the right moment towards the appropriate child. He had a bad limp and I wonder whether he had been wounded in the First World War and could only find employment as a park-keeper. Although it was a worthwhile and useful job, I am sure he was very poorly paid.

Each spring the municipal open-air, unheated, swimming baths opened for the season. The main swimming pool was very large, with a 3ft shallow end for the 'beginners' that gradually deepened to 8ft. 6ins. beneath the diving boards. There was a long chute, separated from a springboard by a range of higher diving boards, with a very high board at the top. It was a large, modern pool, built almost undoubtedly in the early l930s, but now replaced by a large Leisure Centre. There was also a gently stepped paddling pool for the little ones, with a large fountain in the centre. The very sound of the water playing from this fountain was an enticement to step into the pool. On hot summer days this area was always crowded with young children, sitting on the steps as they dabbled their feet in the water, then dashed into the spray under the fountain. They were mostly there with slightly older brothers and sisters. I don't recall many mothers being present. It was, I think, considered a safe place for youngsters to be. What wonderful facilities were provided to encourage all ages in water-sports, but to my knowledge there were no clubs or classes during the War to develop latent talent.

Each spring, on the 1st of May, my friend Joan and I went off to Wealdstone Baths, with five shillings (25p) in our blazer pockets, to buy our book of sixty tickets for the summer season. Our parents paid for these tickets, which enabled us to go swimming during the summer at the price of only one penny (old money) a session. Our pleasures were not costly. The swimming pool was about thirty minutes walk from our home and during the summer we often walked to the baths for a swim after school. The water temperature was chalked up on a board by the turnstile entrance and at the beginning of the season it was only $58°$ or $59°$ F (between $16°$ and $17°$ Centigrade). Our bathes were *very* brief in early May and we swam more for bravado than pleasure in the unheated pool, so that we could boast to our friends and family of swimming in such cold water! As the weather grew warmer we stayed at the baths longer and had great fun jumping into the sparkling water from the concrete surround and making a huge splash, then scrambling out to repeat the performance. Neither of us became accomplished divers, nor were we very proficient at swimming under water, but we enjoyed the satisfaction of improving our swimming strokes, gradually increasing the number of lengths we could do, until we worked out that we swam half a mile. We never had swimming lessons. There was not a children's swimming club to join, nor was there the opportunity of swimming lessons from School. No coaches were available in the War to take children to the Baths. Joan and I swam purely for pleasure in our spare time.

The baths were crowded on hot days during the school summer holidays, and we often spent the entire afternoon in and around the pool, remaining there until the early evening, or until hunger for our tea made us think of home. Steeply raked spectator stands extended along the entire side of the pool and screened the girls' changing cubicles from general view. When warmed by the sun, these green-painted tiers of benches were very welcoming to cold wet bodies after a swim. We spread out our towels to dry on the sun-baked wood and then sun-bathed in our ruched, elasticated, bathing costumes. These were not figure revealing and certainly not figure flattering, but were a great improvement on the hand-knitted affair I had worn when I was little. As we joined all the other children and young people spread along the terraces, we basked in the sun with the sounds of the fountain splashing, jollity and laughter around us, before returning to the water for another dip. It was sheer bliss. I don't remember any bullying or unpleasantness, or ever feeling threatened. There was no hooliganism, and the bathing attendants patrolling around the edge of the pool soon put a stop to any too-boisterous fun, or anyone behaving irresponsibly in the water. Their eyes were everywhere and everyone gave them great respect.

We occasionally treated ourselves to a mug of Bovril from the little refreshment kiosk by the entrance after a swim on a chilly day. This was a rare luxury that warmed us up before we walked home. There was little to buy from the kiosk apart from hot drinks and there were certainly no chocolate bars! The pool was almost empty on cold days; only the enthusiasts (or the foolhardy like Joan and me?) went swimming on a dull, chilly day. The attendants were not so obvious then, were not continually parading around the edge of the almost empty pool, but were sitting in the little ticket office, probably drinking mugs of Bovril too.

One hot Saturday afternoon in 1944 I had gone to the baths on my own. I was contentedly swimming up and down the pool when the air-raid siren blared out its warning of an approaching 'doodlebug' raid. Whistles were blown and everyone was hustled out of the water, out of the changing cubicles and off the sun terraces. The attendants jostled us through a previously unnoticed emergency exit and hastily shepherded us across an adjacent park to the shelters. We had no time to collect our clothes, and everyone ran barefoot across the grass, still in their swimming costumes and into the municipal air raid shelters. There I huddled with all these strangers on the rough benches, damp and dismayed, feeling unhappy, cold and squashed in uncomfortable, unfamiliar surroundings, not even knowing exactly where I was. I felt safe in the shelter but I didn't know the people around me, and I remember sitting there worrying about the safety of my home. I knew there was nobody indoors, but felt afraid that the V1 might drop on our house and that it would be a pile of rubble when I arrived home. After some time the 'All Clear' sounded and with great relief I ran back across the park to the pool, and queued up to exchange the numbered disc that was pinned on my bathing costume for the metal basket that contained my clothes. All I wanted to do was to get dressed and go home as quickly as possible. My fears were unfounded; the house was still standing!

A swimming gala was held at this large open-air pool on the August Bank Holiday following the end of the War. The spectator stands were crowded on this scorching hot afternoon; the dark green paint burned our bottoms when we sat down, but we were all so excited we took no notice. There were various kinds of swimming races: backstroke, crawl, breaststroke, relay, under-water and novelty races (when the competitors dressed up in funny hats or wore pyjamas). The diving displays appeared spectacular to my inexperienced eyes but I recall the greasy pole event most vividly, with the competitors trying to climb the greased pole that was fixed beneath the high diving boards. Almost inevitably they slipped down into the water with a mighty splash, followed by much laughter, shouting and jeering from the excited spectators. It was a good afternoon out. Occasions such as this had not been arranged for years and Joan and I had not seen anything like it before. We didn't have television to provide us with a variety of sporting events to look at. To be a spectator at the swimming gala was a new and exciting experience.

My friend Joan lived in a tree-lined avenue near my home. There was no traffic in Formby Avenue in wartime so the little side road became a wonderful playground where our games were never interrupted by passing (or parked) cars. At the beginning of the War a number of street shelters had been built along one side of the road and their brick walls enabled us to practise and enjoy our many ball games. Our parents would not allow us to bounce our balls against the house walls. Joan's home was pebble-dashed and mine had smooth white walls; our balls would either loosen the stones on her house or mark the white finish on mine. The street shelter was a perfect substitute and we bounced our balls up against its walls in a multitude of different ways as we chanted our rhymes and did the appropriate action with each throw of the ball.

The long brick structure of each air raid shelter was designed to accommodate about fifty people. They were supposedly strengthened and none had been damaged in Formby Avenue, but I have read that they did not withstand much bombardment during the Blitz. During the light evenings of spring and summer we played in the street without a care in the world. We often stood in the middle of the road, throwing the ball to each other over the telegraph wires, which criss-crossed the road to the few homes that were on the telephone. We always seemed to play these ball games during the evenings and never in the daytime. I can sense the quietness as we played together during those evening hours, with a feeling that the road belonged to us. Sometimes another friend joined us and we played 'piggy in the middle' but Margaret was not as agile as we were, didn't throw or catch the ball easily, or move as fast, so she was nearly always the 'piggy'.

Some of the trees in Joan's road bore a crop of small, dark red, decorative, but inedible, fruit. We were making the most of the remaining daylight one summer evening before our outdoor activities were curtailed. We managed to reach up to the branches of one of the trees by the roadside and pulled off some of the little crab-apple-like fruit. They were extremely sour when we bit into them and had a bitter taste, but we pretended to enjoy them. Later on that night we both suffered bad stomach-ache and were sick. We were not well enough to go to school the following day. When we next met and found out that we both been ill, we knew the reason why, but we never informed our families of the cause of our pain and sickness! We had learned our lesson and didn't need anyone to tell us not to repeat the experience or pick the 'forbidden fruit' again.

One winter Joan and I decided to visit the Odeon Cinema on Saturday mornings for the children's picture show. We walked to Kenton High Street and queued up at the box office to pay 3d. (just over lp.) for a ticket for our morning's entertainment. The 'picture house' was packed with children, with the front rows of the stalls already filled with noisy boys who shouted and booed at the 'baddies' and cheered rowdily at the 'good guys' in the cowboy films. After some short cartoon Mickey Mouse and Donald Duck films, the main picture was usually a Western with Roy Rogers (maybe also starring Ronald Reagan?) after which a shorter, second picture usually concluded the morning's programme. It was very good value for 3d. but all I can remember is the wild excitement and shouting of the boys in the stalls and the racket they made. An usherette sometimes marched down the aisle during the showing of a film and shone her little torch at a particularly badly behaved group of boys in an attempt to quell the noise and quieten these rowdies. The usherettes were not quite as expert at controlling the boys in the cinema, as was the park-keeper in the recreation ground, but the threat of being thrown out usually quietened them, but it spoilt our morning's entertainment. I soon stopped going and found something else to do - like queuing for the weekend shopping.

Another of our seasonal pleasures were our expeditions to the woodlands in Stanmore and around Bentley Priory. Harrow & Wealdstone Railway Station was on the main LMS (London, Midland and Scottish) line into Euston. Towards the end of the nineteenth century a short line was constructed from Wealdstone (where the swimming pool was) through to Belmont Station (where we got on the train) and on to, what was then, rural Stanmore. This branch line had been funded largely by a Mr. Frederick Gordon who owned the Gordon Hotel Group. He had acquired the sumptuous mansion, 'Bentley Priory', and converted it into a Hotel. He wanted to provide an easy connection from the main line railway station to Stanmore for visitors staying at the hotel. He had also bought a large area of land for development in Stanmore and the road in which the Stanmore Station was situated was named Gordon Avenue.

In later years the little steam train provided easy access to Harrow & Wealdstone Station for commuters to London from the developing residential areas of Belmont and Stanmore. No doubt the Kodak employees who lived in Stanmore or the Belmont area of Kenton also used it. Good public transport was essential in those days of few car owners, but the 'Belmont Rattler' was one of the many lines that were axed by Dr. Beeching in 1963. Mr. Gordon's Hotel project was not a success, and in 1925 Bentley Priory was purchased by the Air Ministry, and became the Headquarters of Fighter Command during the War.

Joan and I walked up Kenton Lane to Belmont Station and waited for the one-carriage train to take us on the single-track line the short distance to Stanmore. There was one passing place, where we sometimes sat in our compartment, waiting impatiently for the other train to pass by. We had a sandwich in our school satchels for our lunch – nothing fancy, probably Marmite or fish paste! - and our Library books to read in the afternoon. Stanmore Station was built in a Gothic style and looked more like a small village chapel than a railway station. It has now been converted into a private residence. From there Joan and I walked uphill to the rural wooded area around Stanmore Common and Bentley Priory Estate, where, unbeknown to us, Fighter Command Operations Room had been constructed before the War broke out, deep underground, in part of the Estate not open to the public. My husband remembers cycling to Stanmore sometime before the War started and seeing tons of cement being poured into a deep hole in the ground. He didn't know until long after the War was over that this operation was connected with the provision of a bomb-proof Control Centre for Fighter Command.

After exploring different parts of Stanmore Common around the Ponds, climbing trees or roaming around Bentley Priory Woods, we found what we called 'our tree'. We climbed up the old tree until we reached a long overhanging branch, shuffled along it before settling ourselves astride this thick old bough to eat our sandwiches and read our schoolgirl tales. We thought we were having a great adventure; we had no fears; were completely free and independent in the quiet, peaceful place. We had no idea of the time, apart from an innate sense that if the sun began to sink low in the sky, or it began to get a little cool it was time for us to be setting off for home. Maybe hunger pangs also reminded us that it was time for tea. We were unaware of the important Air Ministry activities not far away; we could not see the House, but we occasionally heard the clock chiming faintly in the distance and wondered where the sound came from.

Sometimes we picked hazel catkins, horse chestnut buds, bluebells or blackberries before we went home. I brought 'sticky buds' home in the spring and put them in a vase of water. It was fascinating to see them grow fatter and fatter before they suddenly burst open, showing their bright green leaves and flowers. We all enjoyed the sweet hyacinth smell of the bluebells I carried home from the woods one day, and placed in a vase on the dining table for a brief time before they wilted. One couldn't buy flowers very often in wartime. We picked big bunches of hawthorn blossom one springtime; the delicate pink and white flowers looked so attractive, but Joan's mother would not allow her to bring hers into the house, saying it was bad luck to bring May blossom indoors. There was no such superstition to prevent me from arranging my sprays into vases when I got home, and the heady perfume filled the living room for a day or two, until the blossom drooped and soon dropped all over the floor - perhaps that was the bad luck! In those days one did not understand the necessity of preserving the rural environment and we didn't consider that we were despoiling the countryside by picking a few of these plants amidst the bounty proliferating around us.

Only once did we misjudge the time and left our 'adventure hideout' rather late in the day, not noticing that the sun was already setting as we left our wild wooded area for the lengthy walk to the station. We had to wait a while before the little steam train arrived and gradually we realised that it was twilight and we ought to be home. After the short journey to Belmont Station we were the only two people to get off the train and were probably the only passengers still travelling. We slammed the heavy carriage door shut behind us and hurried to the exit. We were surprised to see Joan's father leaning on his bicycle outside the station, waiting for us, and we recognised by his demeanour that we were in trouble for returning home so late. He was looking agitated and worried, and was very cross. After a ticking off we were told to hurry home as fast as we could, while Mr. Arnett cycled back to tell his wife that we were safe and sound.

We soon encountered my father on his way to the station. He had arrived home from work, discovered my absence and had immediately 'got on his bike' again and was cycling up to the station. Joan's father had warned us that my father would soon be on the 'war-path'. He too looked pretty anxious when we first caught sight of him, so we were quite prepared for our second telling off. I am sure that both our parents were greatly relieved to discover that we had come to no harm. But I don't believe that our fathers were worried in the way that parents would be today, and we certainly had no thought or fear that we could be harmed in any way. I am sure that our families were only anxious that we might have fallen over and sprained an ankle, had some minor accident, or were unaware of the time (which was true), but I have no idea of how they would have begun to search for us if we had had an accident. Stanmore Common and Bentley Priory are pretty large areas of open common land even today.

Children - especially girls - are now unable to go off for the day as we did, unless they are accompanied by an adult, and, most probably, taken by car. There are very few areas in our country now where parents feel that their young people can roam freely without fear of some assault or attack. These risks and fears were not apparent in my childhood. We were not concerned about, or afraid of, or indeed aware of any of the dangers that now have to be explained to children, and in our innocence we enjoyed our unsophisticated pleasures. Our parents were happy for us to explore the nearby countryside and climb the trees. They encouraged our independence, our self-reliance and our freedom. Neither were they afraid we were in any kind of danger. It was a different world! What we did not have in the way of material things - toys, computers or expensive entertainment - we made up for with a far greater measure of liberty.

I spent many hours in my friend Joan's house playing draughts, Snakes and Ladders, Ludo, Old Maid, Rummy, Snap, and other card games that her father had taught her and her younger sister and little brother. I don't remember Joan coming to play at my house. When the weather was too cold to play out of doors we often sat on the living room carpet in her home playing our various games. They kept us occupied and amused while Joan's mother was busy, but whenever possible we were always encouraged to go 'out' to play. Fresh air was good for us!

Her father kept rabbits in cages in the back garden and Joan and I used to stroke these docile creatures, clean out their cages from time to time and give them fresh straw when necessary. Each rabbit had a name and they were like pets to us as we made a fuss of them, but I now realise that they must have been bred for extra meat for the family to supplement their rations. It never crossed my mind at the time that they were anything other than pets, and I never thought that they might sometimes have had rabbit pie for their dinner.

Joan's parents were very good to me, and one Saturday they invited me to join their family on an outing to Harrow Weald Woods. A Saturday excursion was an unusual occurrence for me, as my father was always at work on this day, so it was quite a special treat. We travelled to Harrow Weald on the bus and after a ramble in the woods we went to a nearby pub in Old Redding. We all sat outside in the garden and Joan's parents had a drink. 'The Case is Altered' had a very old-world, rural atmosphere as we sat at a rickety rustic table outside the back of this, now, quite well known public house. Its name is reputedly derived from the name 'Casa Alta' (high house) and some think it was built on the site of a Roman villa. I have no idea how much truth there is in this but there were certainly Roman settlements in the Stanmore area. The pub is situated quite high up, with distant views across London on a clear day. In those days pubs had a very different image from today, and were not generally regarded as places suitable for children. They had no restaurants for family meals, ladies' lunches, snacks, or even coffee, but were mainly for men, drinking, smoking, billiards and darts - and no doubt putting the world to rights, as the customers leaned against the bar.

This was my only experience of a visit to - only the outside of - a pub in my childhood or youth. My father enjoyed a glass of wine or sherry at Christmas time and when he visited our relatives at Mill Hill, but he never went into a public house, and possibly would not have approved of his daughter sitting in the garden of one.

I was given a sturdy, second-hand bicycle for my eleventh birthday. I was soon able to experience the freedom that my bike gave me and enjoyed many cycle rides in the coming years. We called my vehicle a 'sit up and beg' bike as the handlebars were high and my arms were outstretched to reach them. It was quite hard work when pedalling up a hill, as it had no three-speed gears. When I had reached a good speed on a straight, even stretch of empty road, I loved to cycle along with no hands on the handlebars. The empty roads enabled me to enjoy this freedom without having to concern myself with approaching or overtaking cars. Joan was given a bike at around the same time and we soon gave up our train rides to Stanmore and travelled under our own 'steam'.

Few families were able to have many excursions or treats in those days. I never visited a museum in my childhood. (Their treasures had been removed to safer areas for the duration of the War.) There were not many places to go to, as travelling was difficult and entertainment was not the major industry it is today. My father and I were unable to have many outings together because of his working hours. I was free from school on Saturdays when he was working all day and his half-day was on Wednesday when I was hard at work at my lessons. There were no elaborate or expensive family excursions, little opportunity for even modest ones and even less possibility for children whose fathers worked on Saturdays.

However, when I became sufficiently proficient on my trusty (or was it just rusty?) old bike my father and I were able to enjoy a few outings on Bank Holidays and Wednesday afternoons during the school holidays. One August Bank Holiday Monday we cycled to Ruislip Lido, laid our bikes - no padlocks needed! - in front of a hedge and went for a walk in the countryside surrounding the reservoir. As we sat and ate our sandwiches I remember noticing the little blue harebells that were growing in the grass. I can still recall my delight at seeing these dainty flowers, and also my surprise at finding clumps of wild yellow snapdragons nearby, so similar to the antirrhinums I saw in our garden at home. (I think this was the first time that I was aware of wild flowers.) I would now recognise them as toadflax, but I didn't know the names of wild flowers and have never become familiar with the names of many. I could identify antirrhinums, as my father grew the cultivated variety, and we used to have some very handsome specimens in our flowerbeds. Sadly, there are fewer wild flowers, birds or butterflies to be identified or even seen as the years go by. We joined with many other Bank Holiday families as we enjoyed a swim in the Lido.

On another occasion we cycled to Rickmansworth Aquadrome, whistling and calling 'Coo-ee, Uncle Viv' as we pedalled along, as my Uncle Viv (of the beetroot seed 'tease') was then living near Rickmansworth. We didn't know his address, but I foolishly hoped he would hear me calling him as I cycled along. On another Bank Holiday we cycled to Cassiobury Park, an area of open country alongside the canal at Watford, where we cycled along the towpath and had a simple picnic tea by the waterside.

One Wednesday afternoon in my summer holidays we had an oddly memorable excursion to the Thames at Richmond. I went to work with my father in the morning, and after he had closed the shop at I o'clock we set off on a rather dull August afternoon to cycle to Richmond-on-Thames. We crossed the bridge and got on to the towpath, then cycled along for a mile or two by the side of the river. On our return journey along the same track we saw a little makeshift stall had been erected, and behind the improvised counter a man was selling beetroot sandwiches. He had grown the beetroots on his allotment and had made sandwiches with some of his produce. We took advantage of this temporary riverside snack bar and bought two sandwiches – just bread and beetroot. I had never eaten beetroot sandwiches before and I have never eaten them since that day, but they were an off-ration, tasty, colourful treat, and strangely the memory of a beetroot sandwich has not left me. This allotment holder was providing a service with his surplus crop and making a little profit too. These modest outings seem almost bizarre when compared with the variety and opportunity for children's entertainment today, but were seen as great events then and have certainly been remembered in some detail, and with much pleasure.

I was given a more up-to-date second-hand bicycle, with three-speed gears and semi-dropped handlebars, a year or two later and I began to venture further afield on my own. I discovered a beautiful outdoor swimming pool on the other side of Harrow Hill. It had a very different atmosphere from the local one Joan and I regularly visited, with its large paved area around the pool and the painted wooden terraces to sunbathe on. This one had no spectator stands, was probably older, but had attractive, chalet-style changing cubicles with pretty tiled roofs. There were large grassy sunbathing areas at either end of the pool surrounded by groups of flowering shrubs. The pool was situated on the lower slopes of Harrow Hill, and as I swam in it on a hot summer's afternoon, I could see the well-known Hill, with the trees banked up beneath it and the red roofs of houses appearing in between. The famous spire of St. Mary's Church crowned the scene. It was idyllic.

It was quite a long cycle ride to this pool, including a lengthy uphill pull, before reaching the other side of Harrow Hill and I was glad to be able to make use of my lower gears. I didn't go there very often, but it was a delightful place to visit when there was time to spend swimming and lazing around on a Saturday afternoon, or on a sunny summer's day in the school holidays. Occasionally Rose and I went there together. We were very hungry when we arrived home in the evening after our long bike ride home on top of all our swimming, and we hoped that we would find some spare dripping in the larder. We looked forward to our supper snack with much anticipation and raided the larder as soon as we arrived home, hoping to find the jar full, with some to spare that would allow us to tuck in. We relished our supper as we spread slices of bread with the soft, rich dripping, containing all the juices from the previous Sunday's small joint of roast beef, and then sprinkled it with salt before biting into it. I would not dream of eating this nowadays, but it was a wonderful treat at the end of an energetic day in my youth - and saved a lot of our butter and margarine ration!

Meat was much fattier then and even a small piece of beef produced quite a lot of tasty dripping after it was roasted for our Sunday dinner. This was poured off into an old jam jar and used for basting the roast potatoes the following week. The dripping was kept in the larder - not a fridge - so it remained soft and the concentrated natural meat juices in it produced a very savoury jelly. We didn't worry about cholesterol, BSE, or variant CJD, nor did we consider that the dripping might have become contaminated in temperatures of more than the +5 degrees recommended nowadays! We seemed to thrive on it and were never ill.

One summer my father found time to teach me to play tennis on the tennis courts in Kenton Park. We cycled to the large Recreation Ground (where Rose and I had spent our afternoon's absence from Sunday School) on Wednesday afternoons, and he gave me some lessons. My father taught me how to hold my racquet properly, how to serve and how to score. We played the occasional low-key game of tennis together, but he never got to the stage of teaching me how to play a good back-hand stroke, a smash or a lob. Although I used my mother's old wooden-framed tennis racquet, I didn't connect the racquet with her, as I had never seen her playing. The racquet was very heavy and it seemed old-fashioned to me even when I used it as a girl in the nineteen-forties. It had a bulky rectangular wooden press into which I placed the racquet after use. I then had to tighten the big screws at each corner of the press to prevent the frame distorting, or affecting the tautness of the catgut strings. I played tennis with this old racquet until I was given a new one for my twenty-first birthday. I never had the opportunity of having any coaching, knew of no Tennis Club, and did not learn to play tennis at secondary school, so I am grateful for the initial introduction to the game given by my father. When I was in my teen-age years I began to play tennis with my friend Janet, continued playing on and off while my children were growing up, and have enjoyed playing tennis regularly in a local club in my retirement.

In all my various activities with my father, I never considered that there could have been another parent present, or that people might have wondered where my mother was. Other people had mothers but the fact that I lacked my mother's presence never occurred to me. It was in some way blocked out. Nowadays there are so many single-parent families, but Rose and I were the only children I knew at that time who lived with only one parent.

Shortly before beginning my secondary school education I started having piano lessons. I had already been taught the beginnings of musical notation in the recorder group at primary school. We had rather primitive, rudimentary, bamboo recorders on which we had learned to play simple melodies, but the sound we made was rather harsh and reedy. Our housekeeper's daughter had been learning to play the piano with a local piano teacher for some time before I began to have lessons. Mrs. Edgar, who lived nearby, charged 9d. (4p) for a thirty minute lesson. She was a very large, kind-hearted teacher and I enjoyed my lesson with her each week. She was so stout that I used to feel very uncomfortable when my fingers had to reach to the upper register on the piano while playing a piece of music, as my right elbow collided with her solid corporation! I had an Ezra Read tutor book in my early days and learned various simple tunes. 'The Blue Bells of Scotland' comes to mind, but as I progressed I learned a variety of pieces. 'Dusk' by Armstrong Gibbs was a favourite. Rose and I learned and practised all the major and some minor scales and arpeggios, but neither of us took any piano exams and were taught very little musical theory apart from what occurred in the pieces we were studying.

We did our piano practice each day - well, nearly every day - and eventually we were considered to be sufficiently advanced to attempt playing duets together. This was not a good idea! We were endeavouring to play a piano arrangement for four hands of Schubert's 'March Militaire', but as we practised together at home we were continually 'out of step' and could not get it right. We lost our patience, and our tempers, and somehow or other, 'March Militaire' was also mysteriously 'lost'. It was surreptitiously slipped into the dustbin just before the weekly collection, and the dreaded duet disappeared from our lives. Inexplicably - to our respective parents and our piano teacher - the music could not be found when our next lesson was due! I never developed into more than a mediocre pianist, but I have always enjoyed music making and can still play - a little more slowly - some of the pieces I learned when I was young. I find it impossible to learn new works satisfactorily now. It was Mrs. Edgar who suggested that I learned to play Mendelssohn's 'The Bees' Wedding', and one year Rose gave me the music for a Christmas present. This piece is now well beyond my ability. I found it very tricky at the time, but persevered with my teacher's encouragement and think of her when I hear it played occasionally on the radio.

Mrs. Edgar gave a Christmas party for her pupils towards the end of the War. We had coloured paper crackers and wore paper hats, ate sandwiches, cakes and jelly and played simple party games. The spread of food on the table seemed bountiful, but the games appear to me to be very childish now. But childish games used to be enjoyed by children, and it seems sad that life so soon becomes adult and sophisticated for the present generation, who don't experience the innocent pleasures of childhood for very long. The simplicity and innocence of childhood was fun; it passes by so quickly and will never return. We played Pass the Parcel, Musical Chairs and Postman's Knock. This last game resulted in my first kiss, which occurred outside Mrs. Edgar's living room door as a result of the 'postman' choosing my name – perhaps our games weren't so innocent! I was thrilled to bits to hear my name called, but I didn't enjoy the subsequent damp kiss very much! Surely I could not have played such childish games when I was fourteen years of age? I don't know how Mrs. Edgar had managed to provide us with such a sumptuous tea - by the standards of those times – so soon after the War, but it was a party that I really enjoyed. Did she hoard her rations, or had she asked the mothers of her pupils to contribute to the party fare? My piano teacher had no children of her own and her affection and interest were given generously to her pupils.

Shortly after this party I began to learn a piano arrangement of the music from the light operetta, 'Chu Chin Chow'. As a reward for my hard work and modest achievement with this selection of tuneful songs, Mrs. Edgar took me to see 'Chu Chin Chow' when the Wembley Light Operatic Society performed it soon after the end of the War in Wembley (now Brent) Town Hall. I had never been to a live theatrical performance and thought this show was wonderful. I was so sad when she and her husband retired to Devon a year or two later and my piano lessons came to an end. I never heard from her again.

There were no parties, discos, or end of year celebrations at school. Apart from the little party my mother's cleaning lady once took me to and my piano teacher's party, I can only remember one other party during my childhood. A neighbour of ours worked at the huge Kodak Factory at Wealdstone and I was once invited to attend the Kodak Children's Christmas Party. I knew nobody else at this party and felt a little lost. The large hall was full of children, and long tables were set out with food for our tea. We wore paper hats, and after tea there was an entertainment by a professional children's artiste. I may have been to other parties that are long forgotten and feel sure we must have had Sunday School Christmas parties, but I can't remember them and they may not have occurred until the War was over.

We enjoyed family visits to the cinema. 'Auntie' loved the music of Johann Strauss. When the film 'The Great Waltz' was shown at a small cinema in Baker Street, she, Rose and I went up to the West End to see this romanticised tale of his life, which incorporated so many of his waltzes. We all found the light orchestral music very cheering to our spirits, and the tune of 'Tales from the Vienna Woods' was sung and hummed or whistled around the house for many weeks afterwards. When the film came to our local Odeon cinema on general release some months' later we went to see it again and this time my father was able to come with us. It was a very popular film during the War and we saw it three times.

During the interval between the main film and the 'B' movie a magnificent cinema organ used to rise up in front of the audience from below the screen. Multi-coloured lights focused on it from the film projection box. A cinema organist wearing black jacket, white shirt and bow tie sat at the console to entertain us with a selection of light music. The interval was an important part of a visit to the 'pictures' and was always followed by a five or ten minute's film of news about the progress of the War before the second 'B' film began. This was all much more entertaining and interesting than the loud advertisements we have to endure nowadays before the start of a film.

We went to London one Sunday evening to hear Dr. William Sangster, the famous Methodist Minister of Westminster Central Hall. He was preaching at Hinde Street Methodist Church, near Baker Street, because his own Church was badly bomb-damaged. Unnecessary travelling on a Sunday was disapproved of in our church, but 'Auntie' very much wanted to hear Dr. 'Willie' Sangster, as he was affectionately known. He was a highly esteemed preacher and I have a mental picture of a man with a lot of dark wavy hair, who spoke with much verve and vigour. About thirty years later I was surprised to discover that the Principal of the Teacher Training College I attended in Hertfordshire as a mature student was Dr. William Sangster's son.

At some time in my early childhood I had joined the Brownies attached to our new Parish Church. I went to Sunday School at St. Anselm's for a little while, but we had to kneel on the floor to draw our pictures of the story, with our drawing paper resting on the coarse wicker seats of our chairs and I found it so difficult to control my drawing on such a rough base. The chair legs seemed uneven, making the chair wobble and my resulting pictures were pathetic. I so disliked trying to draw that I soon stopped attending the Sunday School, but I was allowed to continue in the Brownies.

I had been put into a 'Six'; I was an 'Elf'. A second-hand, somewhat faded-looking, Brownie uniform dress was procured for me from somewhere. This dress was the cause of my abrupt farewell to Brownies, not because of its faded colour, or its age, but because of its brevity. This was commented on, not by the Brown Owl, or a teacher, but by a group of small boys. One day we had to wear our uniforms to school for a Brownie 'Quiet Day', and as I was walking home some boys called out, "Look at old Sheila Brookie with her knickers showing". I was acutely embarrassed that my dress was so short that my navy-blue knickers were showing! I resolutely refused to wear the dress again and thus cut short my membership of a uniformed organisation. Brevity and bare thighs were not acceptable for young children in those non-permissive days.

I am sure I would have enjoyed life in the Brownies and more especially in the Guides, as I grew older but the opportunity did not come again. We had no uniformed youth organisations at the church I was subsequently taken to. As an only child it would have provided me with company, a variety of social opportunities and interests even in Wartime. I am sure I would have loved the games and activities, working for the badges, camping and the company of other girls. I had joined the Brownies on my own and didn't know any of the other girls who might have encouraged me to continue to attend. It is interesting to consider the little incidents in early life that can have quite an impact on one's future in either positive or negative ways. I should have had the sense to ignore the boys' teasing. Within a few months I would have completely outgrown the old, short dress, and been provided with another, maybe an over-long one, which would have lasted me a long time and kept me in Brownies until I was old enough to join the Guides.

My weekly comic was a treat I looked forward to. Its arrival through the letterbox with the morning paper made it seem very special. I read the Beano from cover to cover every week from the time I received its first issue in 1938. I should have kept these old comics, as they are valuable collectors' items now. A few years later I changed my comic for a girls' magazine called 'Girls' Crystal' and remember that a sparkling hair slide was given away with one of the early editions. I wore this for a while, no doubt thinking I was wearing diamonds in my hair, until one day it slipped off and was lost - my 'diamonds' were certainly not forever! I remember nothing of the contents of 'Girls' Crystal' but it was, I have no doubt, quite devoid of anything of an explicitly (or even covert) sexual nature and probably did not even contain romantic love stories, but schoolgirl tales of boarding-school and midnight feasts and outdoor adventures. We were innocent, guileless and completely unsophisticated by today's standards. We were also free from the teenage pregnancies, temptations, pressures and stresses that the present generation has to deal with, and I am in no doubt as to which period I preferred to grow up in, despite the deprivations and limitations my generation may have experienced.

Cultural visits began at Chandos soon after the end of the War and during our final term, a teacher took a group of girls to one of Sir Malcolm Sargent's Saturday morning Children's Concerts at Covent Garden Opera House. The Opera House was very dirty, dingy and dilapidated and we were quite unimpressed by the war-torn building. We each had to pay 5s. (25p.) for our ticket - a large sum of money for one schoolgirl's entertainment in those days. A year later two teachers at my Commercial College took a group of students to an unforgettable performance of 'The Magic Flute' at Covent Garden on another Saturday morning and the music and costumes were memorable. These special Saturday morning performances for Schools must have been organised with a triple motive: to introduce young people to music and opera; to raise additional money for the restoration of Covent Garden Opera House and they were probably also dress rehearsals for an evening performance. I have never been to Covent Garden since and would dearly love to see a traditional costumed performance of 'The Magic Flute' there. These same two committed and musically enthusiastic teachers also arranged for a group of interested pupils to go to Sadler's Wells Opera House, which looked almost as drab as Covent Garden, to see Madam Butterfly and Tosca. These events were my introduction to the concert hall and opera and were the small beginnings of School cultural trips that later became such an important part of post-war education.

Food shortages made entertaining very difficult and restricted friendships. We did not socialise very much and we certainly never entertained friends to dinner as one does nowadays. I cannot remember eating a meal at my friend Joan's house. Her mother had three children to feed and I think that most mothers wisely kept the contents of their larders for their families. I have no memory of my father or 'Auntie' entertaining friends for a meal and have no recollection of visitors in our home when I was young.

I can't ever remember having a birthday party with games, but do recall having my friend Joan to tea one day, together with another girl, who may have been her sister; maybe this was on my birthday. My main memory of this occasion is linked to the fact that I was suffering from conjunctivitis (or 'pink-eye' as I was told my inflamed, irritated eye condition was called). One of my guests had brought a toy kaleidoscope with her. This was not a present for me, but was her personal possession. I was fascinated with it, peering into the lens to see the ever-changing patterns as I twisted it around. 'Auntie' came into the room and was horrified to see me sitting at the tea table with my infected eye pressed against the end of the tube and gazing down it. She, understandably, was cross with me for being so thoughtless, and took the kaleidoscope away to the kitchen to wash it thoroughly with Dettol, hopefully to remove any germs. I hope the unremembered owner didn't develop conjunctivitis. I never saw a kaleidoscope again until I was an adult and I was even then childishly fascinated by the many patterns that could be produced.

After the little tea party was over I had to have drops inserted into my bad eye before I went to bed. I went upstairs, sat on the bathroom stool and leaned my head back to rest on the towel rail while 'Auntie' put the yellow drops into my eye. She told me to remain there for a few moments so that the medication could spread over my eyeball, and then to get off to bed. But I fell asleep where I was, and was discovered much later that evening, fast asleep on the bathroom stool, with my head still resting on the top of the towel rail. As I grew into my teens this sudden, overwhelming sleepiness used to occur quite frequently. I was alert and awake when on the go and energetic, but sometimes dropped off to sleep suddenly when I was not actively engaged, mentally or physically, in walking, talking, playing, reading, or paying attention to my lessons. It became a little bit of a problem in the evenings when I was at secondary school, as my father sometimes found me asleep over my homework. I wish I could sleep as easily now.

Our main form of entertainment in the evenings was listening to the wireless. We enjoyed 'In Town Tonight' on Saturdays, with the introductory sounds of London's street calls - 'Violets, buy my sweet violets', and 'Star, News or Standard' from flower-seller and newspaper boy (although I cannot recall seeing a flower-seller on the occasions we went up to London) - to the distant accompaniment of traffic sounds. But where would all the traffic have come from in the middle of the War? I always imagined it was driving around Piccadilly Circus; maybe there was some traffic around that now congested junction. Perhaps the sound was purely in my imagination - or caused by my flawed memory? Various famous people who were 'in town tonight' were interviewed and although I was not old enough to be deeply concerned about some of the subjects, I remember that I listened to the programme with interest. It was followed by Music Hall and my father tried - not always successfully - to get home from work before the start of this programme. The various comedy items that were introduced by Jack Warner entertained us all. I particularly remember Elsie and Doris Walters playing the parts of two Cockney friends named 'Gert' and 'Dais' who chatted amusingly about incidents in their lives amongst their supposed neighbours - perhaps a forerunner to Eastenders without the violence, the drugs and the sex? Jack Warner and Elsie and Doris Walters were brother and sisters and I was once told that they had lived near my parents when they were young. 'Happidrome' was a regular fixture, with its signature tune, "We three, at Happidrome, working for the BBC, Ramsbottom, and Enoch and me", and brought us all to sit around the fire in the evening and enjoy an hour of laughter. I don't recall who Ramsbottom, or Enoch, or 'me' were played by.

I always enjoyed listening to Harry Hemsley impersonating all the voices of his imaginary family of young children, one of whose garbled speech he could never understand. ITMA was another popular programme, with Tommy Handley's quick wit and the regular sayings of "Can I do you now, sir?" and "I've brought this for you" from his 'Mrs. Mopp'. We also enjoyed Arthur Askey in 'Bandwagon' with his regular introduction of "Hello, playmates" followed by the well scripted, but apparently spontaneous, humour throughout the programme. He cheered everyone's lives with his comical songs - 'I'm a bee, a busy, busy Bee' - but I doubt whether these programmes would appear amusing now.

Some of these comedy programmes occurred after I was supposed to be asleep. Sometimes I got out of bed and crept down the stairs, hoping they wouldn't creak and give me away as I sat on the staircase, hidden behind the solid banister. My ears were pricked, trying to catch the words of the jokes, but having to smother my laughter in case I was heard. I am sure that none of the humour was overtly offensive, blasphemous or obscene and was enjoyed by all ages. Anything in questionable taste would have been disguised by a *double entendre* and younger listeners would not have comprehended the alternative meaning. Censorship and the different standards of family life, obscenity and morality then, made it unlikely for the BBC or filmmakers to corrupt children in any way, or debase society, nor were there advertisements on commercial airwaves or channels to exploit them. It was not an 'I want' society. There was no TV.

We hurried home from church on Sunday evenings to listen to the Palm Court Orchestra playing light music from Torquay - near to where my Aunt and Uncle were evacuated. Was it really from Torquay, I wonder now? Did we really have time to listen to the Palm Court Orchestra, Sunday Half Hour, and the Classic Serial on the same evening, after we had walked to the evening Service and then walked home again afterwards? Time must have passed more slowly long ago! On Monday evening another programme was eagerly awaited; this was 'Monday Night at Eight', introduced by Ronnie Waldman and incorporated 'Puzzle Corner'. We enjoyed 'Henry Hall's Guest Night' and Reginald Dixon playing the organ from the Ballroom at Blackpool, and later on Victor Sylvester and his dance band was very popular, with his soft voice of instruction, "Slow, slow, quick, quick, slow....".

'Music While You Work' was broadcast every morning for the factory workers and those at home, and 'Children's Hour' at teatime. A little more serious, but usually entertaining and listened to attentively, was the Radio Doctor, who gave weekly recipes and hints for healthy living in his deep plummy voice after the morning news bulletins. These programmes cheered, entertained and brightened the lives of so many factory workers, families, children and those living alone during that period.

It is a tribute to the Directors, Programmers and Artistes at the BBC during my childhood that I can still remember so many of the programmes they broadcast all those years ago. I wonder which of the present day programmes, presenters, comedians, or stars on radio and television will be equally well remembered in sixty to seventy years' time? The radio was our constant form of entertainment, summer and winter, and must be considered one of the paramount interests throughout my entire my childhood.

Chapter Fifteen

NEW BEGINNINGS

I began my secondary education in the autumn of 1942 and found that, like my primary School, Chandos School was also split into two separate institutions, sharing the same site as a single two-storey building. One was Chandos Senior Girls' School, and the other was Chandos Senior Boys' School. The two schools were being built during the period leading up to the War, and they opened on August 29th, 1939. They functioned for less than a week before being instructed to close after the War was declared on September 3rd. Both schools reopened after Christmas, giving only part-time education for pupils for a further period before full-time lessons began again. Chandos School(s) never had an official Opening Ceremony.

There were only nine teachers in the Girls' School when it first opened, but the all-female staff had increased by the time I began my secondary education in 1942. Miss Pike, the first Headmistress, was greatly respected, and influenced many girls who passed through her School. She was gentle in manner, yet firm; kind, but expecting high standards of behaviour from her pupils both on and off the School premises; serious in her demeanour, but with a humorous twinkle in her eye and a heart-warming smile. She put her stamp on the School from its inception, with her devotion to it and to her pupils. High standards of work, morality, behaviour and consideration for others were subtly instilled in her pupils.

My old School has now been renamed Park High Comprehensive and is a large co-educational School. Its initial (and continued) good reputation was praised by the Mayor of Harrow in her speech at the Diamond Jubilee celebrations of Chandos (now Park High) School in 1999. There has been much restoration and modernisation of the original buildings in recent years and new Departmental Blocks have been built for the requirements of twenty-first century education. How different is the education system today from that of sixty years ago! We had no well-equipped Art, Technical or Science Departments, no Drama or Music Departments, no large well-stocked Library, no Sports Centre (although we were very proud of our Gym, which has now been replaced by a large Sports Hall). Of course, we had no computers and knew nothing about Information Technology! We were not encouraged, or expected, to have opinions in our lessons, to make judgements, discuss our work either with our teacher, each other, or in a group. There were no school plays, prize-giving ceremonies, end of term concerts, or dances (discos were unheard of); no school excursions, educational holidays, consultation evenings or cultural visits. Our experience at Covent Garden in our final term was particularly memorable because it was the first School trip after the end of the War.

I remember only one 'Open Afternoon' that was arranged just before the end of my third and final year, when parents were invited to the School to see our work. My father could not attend a School function during the daytime so our housekeeper came instead, and sat at my desk looking through my exercise books, in which all our written work was done. She read one of my 'Compositions' and chatted to the mother of the girl who sat next to me. There was no elaborate display of our work to look at on the walls of the corridors or classrooms and as far as I can remember, no opportunity was given to talk to my form mistress. My father never saw the inside of either my Junior or my Senior School because we never had an Open Evening.

The School is situated on a small hill about a mile away from my old home, with pleasant, open parkland leading up to it. During the War some of this open space and also our school field was used by nearby householders for allotments to grow their own fruit and vegetables. Laing's, the large building Company, built a large development of semi-detached houses in the area during the l930s. What had in earlier times been the hamlet of Kenton and the village of Stanmore were vastly extended to become a part of suburbia, producing the necessity for new schools. The Laing's Construction

Company probably built the School too. It had a wide catchment area and took pupils from eight primary schools. There was no parental choice of Senior School; children were allocated to the one nearest to their home.

I called for my friend Joan on the morning of our first day at Senior School, and I had also knocked on the door of another girl who sometimes used to play ball with us in the street. She had been in my primary school class. Margaret was nervous about going to the 'big' school, and her mother had knocked on our door to ask if I would call for her daughter. We three girls set off together feeling self-conscious, but rather proud of ourselves in our new uniforms, walking through the streets then up the hill through the park to our new school. New pupils had no opportunity of visiting the school before this important first day of term, so we were in completely unfamiliar surroundings. No doubt we all felt a little apprehensive as we joined the other new girls who were beginning a fresh stage in their lives.

We sat cross-legged on the fine parquet floor of the large school Hall, waiting to be assigned to our respective classes; any girls we knew from our Primary School were lost in a sea of strange faces. We were in a very different kind of building from our previous wooden school, with its small hut-like assembly Hall. This Hall accommodated several hundred people and had a large raised stage approached by a number of steps each side. A table was placed in the middle of the stage, with an impressive grand piano to one side. We looked up at our new Headmistress as she addressed us from her elevated position. She welcomed us, explained the rules of the School and briefly described the House system. Each girl was then allocated to one of four Houses: Stanmore, Canons, Whitchurch and Brockley. We were later given coloured badges to pin on to our gymslips to denote to which House we belonged. Stanmore was red, Canons blue, Whitchurch white and Brockley was green. I was placed in Brockley House.

The family name of Chandos existed at the time of William the Conqueror, and a descendent was created Duke of Chandos early in the eighteenth century. He married into the family who owned Canons, in the Manor of Whit Church (Whyt Church being an early descriptive name of the Church attached to the Manor). It had been in existence since the twelfth century and is mentioned in the Domesday Book. The name 'Canons' came about because much land in the area had been given to the Priory of St. Bartholomew's in Great Smithfield, London. Many Canons from this Priory had been involved in the estate before the Dissolution of the Monasteries and so it acquired the name 'Canons'.

During the eighteenth century the Duke of Chandos was appointed Paymaster General to the Duke of Marlborough, and acquired vast estates in Canons and Little Stanmore, near Edgware, not far from the old Great North Road (now Al) and so was within easy reach of London by stagecoach. He amassed a fortune during the period and had a huge mansion built, named Canons, where he entertained the elite in Society. Handel was attached to the household for some years, and played the organ at the baroque Church of St. Lawrence's, WhitChurch, before he moved elsewhere and began composing opera and his famous oratorios. The Chandos Anthems were composed here and so named in honour of his patron. The Church has been restored and its interior is still beautiful.

The Duke of Chandos lost much of his wealth through his extravagant living and had to break up his Estate to pay off his enormous debts, and Canons soon lost its social importance. The large Mansion was demolished and parts sold off for use in large estate Houses elsewhere. A smaller Georgian house was subsequently built upon the site. Some of the Estate remains as a public open space.

In 1929 the famous North London Collegiate School for Girls bought Canons House and some of the adjoining land, moving from Camden in North London to its present site in Canons Park, and there developed the present large, modern, highly regarded Independent School. Although it was a move to a rural area at the time, urbanisation and the spread of Greater London has led to the present North London Collegiate School being situated once more in the northern outskirts of the Capital. Some years later Harrow Urban District Council (now part of Greater London Council) acquired much land in the area – St. Bartholomew's or Canons Estate land? - no doubt anticipating future development.

Brockley is the name of a hill in Stanmore and is possibly part of the old Canons or Great Smithfield Priory land. The well-known National Orthopaedic Hospital is situated at the top of Brockley Hill, but it was known as Brockley Hospital when I was young. Brockley has an even older history than the other three School Houses. It was known as Sulloniacae and was a Roman staging post nine miles from Verulamium (St. Albans), on the route known as Watling Street that runs from Richborough in Kent to Hadrian's Wall in Northumberland. Only now do I understand the background of the name given to the School Houses, the School and the history of the area around which it was built.

My old School is possibly built on some of the land within the boundaries of the original Estate of the Duke of Chandos, or land that had previously belonged to the Priory of Great Smithfield. It seems a pity that we were not taught the significance of the name of our School or the history of the area whilst we were pupils. The names of our School Houses would have had more meaning if we had known the relevance of their background. What interest it would have added to our history lessons, and I am sure it would have enthused some of us to research further into our local history.

Chandos pupils may not have had the status, the intellectual ability, the high level of academic attainment, the wealthy parents, or the opportunities of nearby North London Collegiate School pupils, but I believe that the Headmistress of my own School was as equally dedicated to girls' education as the well-known educationalist Dame Kitty Anderson, who was then Headmistress of the girls' Public School not very far away from my more lowly Senior School. At the time I had never heard of North London Collegiate.

After our initial introduction to the ways of the school, individual teachers called out the names on their registers, and lines of girls filed out of the Hall in silence to their new form rooms. Although I had been extremely disappointed that I had not achieved my ambition of going to the County School, I already felt happier about the atmosphere, and perhaps sensed the dedication in my Senior School, and my inner shame subsided a little. Margaret, whom I had called for earlier in the morning, and I, were placed in the same class, but sadly my long-standing and close friend Joan, was assigned to a different form. We remained friends, still went to school together, played together, went swimming and continued to have our outings and excursions in holiday times, but saw little of each other during the school day. Margaret and I were both fair-haired, were of similar build and sat next to each other in class. Comments were sometimes made at first that we looked like twins, but we were very unlike in our personalities and did not become close friends with each other despite having been thrown together by circumstance. In our first year (Year 7) we shared a double desk in the row beside the windows. There were five rows of desks, all facing the blackboard that extended the entire width of the front of the classroom - and most importantly - we faced our form teacher.

We all feared, revered, respected or adored Miss Oyston, but not all those emotions were experienced at the same time, or by the same girls! She was a good teacher, who had no difficulty in controlling her large class of forty-six pupils. She was strict, but with a sense of humour and kindliness. She was always in command of her class, taught us well and we heeded her words. She had to be firm to control forty-six girls. The whole school was 'streamed' and Miss Oyston's was form teacher of IA, the top stream.

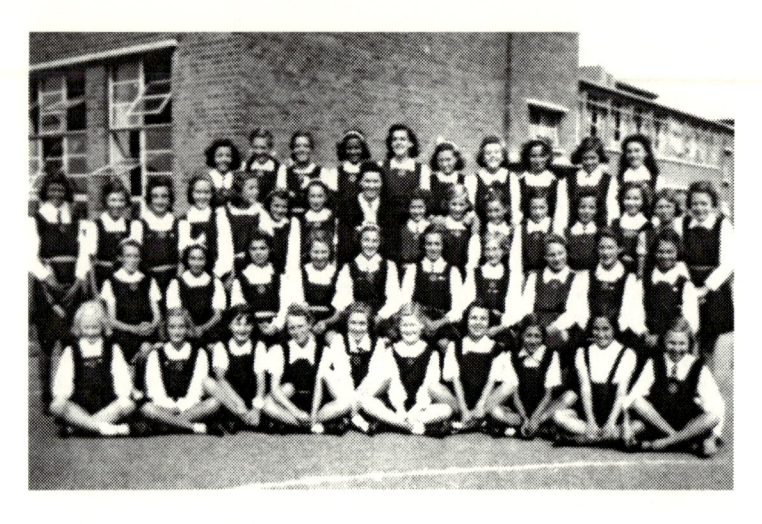

Form 1A (I am last on the right in the bottom row!).

There was no contact with the boys who occupied the other half of the School building. A clear, white dividing line was painted across the playground, separating the boys' School from the girls', and we were not allowed to step over the line. Break periods were taken at different times, with the exception of the dinner hour, when some fraternisation occasionally occurred. I was not at all interested in the boys' half of the playground, with the noisy shouts arising from their rough, informal games of football. We shared the gymnasium that was situated at the boys' end of the School, but timetabling ensured that we never met any boys as we walked silently in single file through their part of the School to our gym lessons. Any association with the opposite sex was unlikely, strongly discouraged and officially forbidden. Our class 'crocodile' to the gym each week did not spark any curiosity. I always thought the boys' end of the School building looked dirtier and scruffier than our end. After I left Junior School, boys became an almost non-existent species in my childhood experience.

Our curriculum was very restricted, partly because we were not in a Grammar School but also because we must have been very far behind in our studies. We had lost a large chunk of our basic education because of the school closures at the beginning of the War and had further interruptions during the Blitz, when we had spent hours in the air raid shelters. Our School was not fully equipped when it opened just before the War. There was only one Art Room, with very few facilities; a Science room, with benches and stools, but without any equipment; a tiny school Library was housed in part of a disused classroom but there were very few books on the shelves, we rarely entered the room, and never consulted any reference books to help us gain additional information for any of our lessons. Wartime produced a shortage of paper and consequently a shortage of books. The present large School Library is very impressive, with a good collection of books on many subjects filling its shelves and bays. What a contrast with the l940s!

Chandos School may also have been understaffed. We did not have specialist teachers for each subject and there were no graduate teachers in the girls' school (and only two graduates in the boys' school) when it opened. Very few girls in the twenties or thirties went to University. Those who did gain a degree and wanted a career in teaching would have been unlikely to take up posts in Senior Schools. There were no 'special needs' teachers.

Until the l944 Education Act began to be implemented after the War, basic secondary education lasted only three years, and Senior School pupils could leave as soon as they reached the age of fourteen. It had not entered my head at the age of eleven what I might want to do in the future. I am sure that most of my classmates lived for the present, and we were just hoping to enjoy our schooldays. The burden of study, thoughts of further education, aspirations of future careers and the pressures surrounding the present generation of school students were not our experience.

On arrival at school each morning we usually played 'he' or other active games in the playground until the teacher on duty rang the school hand-bell vigorously. Class numbers were called out and girls filed silently into the cloakrooms. For a few minutes bedlam reigned as we scrambled through the crowd to find our coat pegs. Rows of numbered pegs were fixed above long wooden benches and the named, coloured, check-patterned gingham plimsoll bags (made in our needlework lesson) that hung on each peg, helped to identify the exact location of our possessions. The smell of our rubber-soled plimsolls permeated the cloakrooms and was augmented on wet or wintry days by our rubber, knee-high, Wellington boots and damp, gabardine raincoats. (Wet playtimes or dinner hours were spent in the cloakrooms, sitting and chatting, cramped together on the benches, or squatting on the floor playing our usual pencil and paper games.) A long, heavy iron grille was dragged across the entire front of the cloakroom area after registration each morning and afternoon, and securely locked. Property went 'missing' occasionally but we did not have to carry all our personal belongings around with us every day, and more items were mislaid through carelessness than were deliberately stolen. My brown leather satchel (a birthday present from my father) contained my homework - but no snacks, biscuits or sweets – and we kept most of our other books in our desks, which had lift-up lids. We had little in the way of personal possessions to cram into our satchels or desks. Homework was set each day but it was not unduly onerous.

We soon learned more of the School rules. House Marks were awarded for especially good work, but if anyone behaved badly they risked getting a 'warning Mark'. If three 'warning marks' were collected during a month, a House Mark was lost. This was considered a terrible disgrace. At the end of each month the 'good' House Marks were added up for each respective House and the 'bad' marks were deducted. The House with the highest marks had the honour of having a broad silk ribbon in the appropriate colour tied around the School Shield for the following month. There was keen competition to win the greatest number of House Marks for good work and behaviour and to have the coloured ribbon of one's House tied around the Shield for the following four weeks. The Shield had pride of place on a table in the School Entrance Hall. It, was brought into Assembly in the School Hall by the Head Girl and placed on the table from where Miss Pike addressed us. We developed a fierce loyalty to our particular House. At the end of the School Year all the marks gained were added up and the winning House had its name engraved on to a smaller shield, which was then permanently affixed, to the large School Shield.

Our teachers marked our class work meticulously, and any errors had to be corrected, and grammatical or spelling mistakes were written out correctly three times. Marks were given and House Marks earned for exceptionally good work. We wondered what the Christian names of our teachers were when they initialled a comment or awarded a House Mark, (especially our Form Teacher, Miss Oyston's, 'EGO'). We thought and greatly prized any encouraging or complimentary comment written by her at the end of a piece of work. These comments encouraged us to do our best and to play our part in helping 'our' House to have its ribbon on the Shield the following month. 'Warning Marks' were handed out for talking, running in the corridor, rudeness or disobedience. If the dreaded three Warning Marks had been received during one month, the culprit had to go to Miss Pike's office to report this grave offence, where she was given a serious reproof and the House Mark was officially deducted. This was considered a terrible disgrace. She also received the displeasure of other members of her House for letting them down. The system did keep us 'on our toes', taught us loyalty to a group and encouraged us to work to the best of our ability. Occasional very bad behaviour was punished by the immediate loss of an entire House Mark. This was a rare occurrence and considered a great dishonour to both House and the School.

In recent years I have had the pleasure of getting in touch with a number of my old classmates, and on our first meeting together after almost fifty years, we reminisced about our school days. Vera remembered the occasion when she had already collected two warning marks in one month before being caught talking in the corridor by a teacher. She was told to go to the particular teacher's room to have this black mark recorded. This would have meant a meeting with Miss Pike and the loss of a House Mark. Vera would have been 'on the carpet'! She recalled that it was near the end of the month, so she delayed the collection of her third warning mark until the following Monday. A new month would have begun and she thus avoided the disgrace of a lost House Mark. I remember Vera as a very 'good' girl and cannot imagine that she could ever have been in such danger. She must have been very unlucky that month. She didn't sail so close to the wind again!

Jean recalled the occasion when she was told to leave the class by an irate Miss Oyston because she had giggled at her friend, Faith's, little joke. Jean, being a 'sparkly' girl with a sense of humour, couldn't help responding to the joke, but she was blamed; Miss Oyston's finger was pointed at her, and with the command of 'Out', she left the room and stood in disgrace outside the classroom door until the end of the period, feeling the unjustness of her punishment. She didn't complain, but she has remembered the incident over a period of well over fifty years!

Another friend who subsequently gained an Honours Degree in Australia as a mature student wrote to me with some remembrances of her days at School. She remembered the day she and her friend, Joy, skipped the needlework lesson they loathed (as did I) and hid in the air raid shelters. They were both tomboys and full of high spirits. As the lesson proceeded they crept out of the gloomy shelter, and in their elation at their moments of freedom they began to leap daringly from the top of one shelter to another. A teacher glanced out of her first floor classroom window and spotted them. They were called in and sent straight to the Headmistress, where they stood with quaking knees before Miss Pike, who told them how disappointed she was in them.

My friend still remembers how ashamed she felt, and tells me that they both felt they had disgraced their House and their School. She has never forgotten the incident and even now doesn't want her name revealed! Her subsequent academic and career successes don't equate with her being either a 'Scholarship' failure or a discredit to her old school! Both she and I sadly lost touch with irrepressible Joy. The stories give examples of the standard of behaviour expected of us in those days. These misdemeanours are amusing and almost absurd in retrospect, but they seemed very grave and of great importance at the time.

On one occasion a girl played truant and left the school premises for an entire afternoon. This was unheard-of, and the whole school was informed in our special Friday afternoon Assembly about this serious misdeed. Miss Pike seemed very solemn, obviously saddened and shocked that the girl in question could so disgrace herself and the School. We learned that she was caned across her hand. Until then corporal punishment had been unheard of in our Senior School experience (although I remember once having to hold my hands out and was hit with a ruler in my Infant School because I had talked in class). We were not told who the girl was, but it was a subdued crowd of girls who left the premises that afternoon, and no one else played truant while I was at the School.

Yet in her severity over these individual shortcomings, I believe Miss Pike was still gentle. Although I was never at the receiving end of any reprimand from her (apart from a lapse in my grammar when speaking to her on one occasion!) and cannot speak from experience, I feel sure she spoke to the miscreant with sternness, combined with kindness, in an endeavour to improve attitude and behaviour, to induce responsibility for personal actions, consideration and loyalty to others.

The School took pupils with varied abilities from different backgrounds, but, apart from some occasional bad behaviour from a few girls, there was an overall sense of self-control, pride in the school and respect for the teachers. I only remember kindness from my teachers, who had an easy ability to maintain class discipline and keep our interest. Sometimes their teaching was mixed with a little humour, but there was no over-friendliness or informality and one or two members of staff were very strict. At the time they seemed to be very mature - or almost elderly - but I now realise that most of them were quite young and possibly inexperienced.

Our morning break-time was still preceded by the free provision of one-third-of-a-pint of full-cream milk, which we still drank from a small bottle with the aid of a straw. Semi-skimmed milk was not then available (other than in tins of Nestlé's sweetened condensed skimmed milk). Our daily bottles of milk had a good head of cream above the white, less rich milk. As our School was centrally heated we had none of the problems of icy milk during the winter - nor were we ever sent home because of icy classrooms in our modern, centrally heated school – but the radiators were not always warm.

Our playtimes, or break periods, still seemed to follow an imperceptible routine of games for different seasons of the year. We still enjoyed skipping games and ball games and became very proficient at 'five stones'. 'Dipping' was often a preliminary activity, deciding who would be the leader of a game or a member of a team. Girls were gradually eliminated, or selected, depending on the purpose of the 'dip', but the 'dip' itself often became the game! 'Hic, Hac, Hoc' was popular, and the words with their accompanying hand actions portraying scissors, stone and paper were used in one of our playground 'dips'. (At the time I didn't know that Hic, Hac, Hoc, was a little bit of Latin. I have never understood what it meant! We were not taught Latin, unlike our unknown contemporaries in North London Collegiate School at nearby Canons Park.)

The two winners of Hic, Hac, Hoc, became the leaders, who picked their teams, choosing the best runners, best throwers or catchers first. Each girl was carefully considered for her ball skills and speed and there was always a great sense of pride if one was chosen early on in this selection process. A game we called 'Kingie" was very popular and was prepared with bits of rough wood that were carefully balanced in a particular manner against the playground wall. When the teams had been picked, the two leaders would 'dip it out' to decide who played first. This team then took it in turns to throw a small ball at the crude wooden framework propped up again the wall until it was gradually knocked to the ground. The girls scattered and spread out in the playground and the second team had possession of the ball. They threw it to one another until someone was close enough to hit one of the opposition with it. She was then 'out'. Gradually the rest of the team was eliminated and the opposing side had its innings. It was energetic and exciting and kept us out of mischief during the long, cold dinner-hour in the winter. It was very popular and often continued through several playtimes, but I have never met anyone else who played this game. Did we make up the rules ourselves?

We seemed to spend all our spare time in active games and didn't chat to one another about personal matters at all. Friendships were not as intimate as young people's friendships appear to be today. We did not share thoughts, exchange confidences, hug each other, or talk about personal matters, our families, or our aspirations - if we had any.

Most girls had their mid-day dinner at school. Many mothers were at work and would be relieved to know that their children were getting their main meal at school, which helped out with the rations. Only a comparatively few girls with younger brothers or sisters at home, whose mothers were not working, and who lived near enough to the School, were able to go home at dinner-times.

As mid-day approached the caretaker set up wooden trestle tables in the School Hall. Dinner ladies then laid the tables while we all queued up at the small kitchen hatch for our meal. There was no menu, no choice of food. We tried to find a place at a table with our friends, carrying our plate of food carefully across the Hall. A dinner monitor sat at the head of each table and was responsible for the good behaviour of those sitting around her. Grace was always said before our meal, 'For what we are about to receive may the Lord make us truly thankful. Amen'. Some of the staff sat at a table on the stage, the 'high table', eating their meal with us, but above us and facing us. We were not unduly conscious of their presence, but if the noise level became too high, a teacher's voice was sometimes heard over the din, ordering us to be quiet. Hopefully, the fact that some of the Staff were able to gaze down upon us had the necessary calming effect on any unduly raised chattering voices, but nevertheless it was still quite noisy in the School Hall at dinner time and I am sure (from my own subsequent experience) that the teachers disliked being on 'dinner duty'.

Spam was served frequently, in fritters or cold with salad. I was not so keen on the Spam but I enjoyed the salad, which was a mixture of finely chopped cabbage, onion, grated carrot and chopped beetroot, which gave it a wonderful deep red colour. Lettuce and tomatoes were only available in the greengrocer's in the summer season and neither of these salad ingredients came within the budget of school dinners.

We had plenty of filling puddings: spotted dick with custard (suet pudding with a few currants in it), steamed jam sponge with custard, semolina pudding with a blob of red jam in the middle, rice pudding, jam tart and custard. Tapioca pudding was usually greeted with noises of distaste and, with it's' rather slimy, frog-spawn-like consistency, was generally considered inedible, but I liked it. Jam seemed to feature with almost every pudding and custard was nearly always served. We very rarely, if ever, had a pudding with fruit in it and fresh fruit was never available. My favourite pudding was chocolate roll with chocolate sauce. Our housekeeper didn't use cocoa in cooking and I had always found my Auntie Connell's chocolate cakes and chocolate blancmange much to my taste and had a similar passion for school chocolate pudding. I was more than happy to finish off some of my friends' portions; they thought this pudding was horrible and turned up their noses at it! I should have got fat as I hastily devoured my supplementary slices of chocolate roll before the plates were cleared away, and we were sent out into the playground to continue with our game of 'Kingie'.

Chapter Sixteen

LESSONS FOR LIFE

Our Senior School curriculum contained a slightly wider range of subjects than we had been taught in Junior School. I think we all enjoyed Domestic Science lessons, as we were able to move around in the spacious, bright kitchens while we performed our various domestic procedures, instead of sitting at our desks in the classroom. It was a completely new experience to use the modern gas stoves that had been installed when the School had first opened. These were more up-to-date than the cookers most of us had at home. We were taught how to prepare everyday dishes in these well-equipped kitchens, and our Domestic Science course also included such mundane things as housewifery and mending.

We had a mixture of mainly practical lessons, but learned little about food values, vitamins, carbohydrate and protein requirements, or health, hygiene and safety in the home and kitchen. We were less interested in our occasional theoretical lessons; it was the excitement and anticipation of preparation, followed by the satisfaction of a tasty (or just plain edible) result from our cookery lessons that we relished. The necessity of fresh fruit and vegetables in our diet was not emphasised. There was little fresh fruit available and certainly no exotic, unseasonable, imported vegetables. Nevertheless, I think the necessity of eating plenty of vegetables was taken for granted and was certainly highlighted in the Radio Doctor's weekly broadcasts, where vegetables were recommended in all kinds of guises and recipes, from carrot jam to potato pie.

The week before our cookery lesson we were given a list of ingredients that we had to procure from home. It must have been difficult for our teacher, Miss Pearce, to devise suitable recipes, using ingredients that would not cause the family rations to be unduly plundered - particularly if the consequent dish turned out to be a disaster. It was equally hard for mothers to relinquish the ingredients required for, hopefully, a palatable meal, to be prepared, cooked and carried safely home. But the necessary items were found, alternative ingredients were substituted for whatever was unobtainable and the recipe was prepared and cooked. We made vegetable soup, baked potatoes in their jackets with a savoury, cheesy filling. We baked small cakes, beating the ingredients together with a fork and turning them into 'butterfly cakes' by removing the tops and cutting them in half to make 'wings'. More hand beating of hard margarine and sugar produced a 'mock' butter cream, a blob of which was put on each cake, topped off with a pair of 'wings'. Chopped up prunes were used as a substitute for currants in little fruitcakes. In one lesson we attempted to make Chelsea buns, using yeast, with, I seem to recall, a somewhat shapeless, heavy, doughy result. My cheese croquettes were much more successful and I proudly took them home for tea. When they had been reheated, they were very tasty and I made them many times after my initial attempt at school. We were even expected to bring a small joint of beef to school one week, together with some potatoes and in our afternoon cookery session we prepared and cooked a roast 'Sunday' dinner.

In addition to our cookery classes we learned how to clean the small demonstration 'flat' that was part of our Domestic Science Department. We were shown how to lay a table correctly and a select group of girls was once chosen to entertain some of the staff to a meal in this 'flat'. Darning was another of the simple household skills we learned to do in our Domestic Science lessons. We were required to attain an almost professional standard of invisible mending, using threads teased out from an obscure part of the fabric of a garment to repair a small tear in such a way that it really was almost impossible to detect.

Some achievement in my Domestic Science lessons seems to be confirmed by my D.S. teacher's comment in an old school report, although I have no idea how 'Very Good' or 'Neat and thoughtful work' could possibly relate to the periods we spent being shown how to wash clothes by hand in the large sinks beneath the windows. This was certainly not the kind of vocational training we were interested in - unless any of us wanted to go into service or become laundry-maids!

However some of the principles and techniques learned in school cookery lessons were an asset to me as I grew up and I have always enjoyed cooking and serving appetising, nutritious meals. My subsequent satisfaction in cooking was also encouraged through sitting at the kitchen table watching our housekeeper making cakes or pastry and helping her with the cooking. My initial interest may have started even earlier than this when I was living away from home, observing my elderly Aunt's maid, Olwen, as she went about her work in the kitchen.

If more emphasis had been placed on teaching some of these skills to school pupils in recent years perhaps we would not have a generation of young people growing up with little practical knowledge of how to cook nourishing, economical meals. So many appear to live on expensive fast food, pre-packed and micro waved meals, snacking and grazing, or eating out in restaurants (and as a consequence suffer from malnutrition or overweight). Children learned a lot about basic cooking years ago through watching and helping their mothers about the house and in the kitchen. Despite all the modern labour-saving devices that are taken for granted today, many mums seem to have little time to prepare a home-cooked meal. Many families rarely seem to experience the pleasure of sitting around the table together, sharing in a home-cooked meal. The television, the computer, the mobile phone and the Internet seem to have taken the place of the family meal table.

Scripture heads the list of subjects on all my Senior School reports, although apparently it was not considered necessary to be included in our exams, as no mark, grade or comment is given. In each of my three annual reports there is a blank space beside this subject heading. We did have regular lessons based on the Bible in what was then termed Religious Knowledge, but knew nothing about other religions, either from our day-to-day experience, or through our religious education. My First Year (now called Year 7) form mistress, Miss Oyston, was a geographer, and she made the most of St. Paul's first, second and third missionary journeys in her Scripture lessons. The maps we drew and outlined, the dotted lines indicating each route of Paul's three voyages, the incidents, adventures and churches he founded in each city, are the parts I most easily remember. It was rather like a topic in a geography course.

In our Second Year, we had the story of Moses in the bulrushes, studied the life of the Israelites in captivity in Egypt and their eventual escape; the wanderings in the wilderness and their journey to the Promised Land. Our form teacher was Jewish and this helped to make our Old Testament R.K. lessons particularly interesting. She had married shortly before we went into her class and her name changed from Miss Lewonski to Mrs. Humphries during our summer holiday. Her husband was in the Forces and was posted to the Middle East almost immediately after her marriage, and in one lesson she read out to us part of a letter he had written to her describing the desert landscape. We considered what the manna from heaven might have been that appeared each day for the Children of Israel in the wilderness, and discussed the possible reasons why the plagues occurred in the particular sequence referred to in the Old Testament.

We had to memorise the Ten Commandments in our Third Year and I can recall standing at the back of the classroom between two rows of desks while reciting the complicated Authorised Version from Exodus Chapter Twenty, and receiving a coveted House Mark at the end of the successful recitation. I can still recite them! I wonder how many young people today would even know where the Ten Commandments are to be found.

In our last term at Chandos we were required to learn from memory the famous thirteenth chapter from the first book of Corinthians in the New Testament, in which the Authorised Version uses the word 'charity' instead of 'love'. "Though I speak with the tongues of men and of angels and have not charity (love), I am become a sounding brass or a tinkling cymbal... now abideth these three; faith, hope and charity, and the greatest of these is charity". We did not fully comprehend what we were memorising, but a little of the meaning of this passage must have rubbed off on to some of us and was understood more as we grew more mature in our own thinking. I am sure that our Headmistress was anxious that none of her pupils should leave the School without knowing the Ten Commandments, or having the chapter about self-sacrificial love and concern for others stored away in their minds. How much more would we have understood of these parts of the Bible if a modern translation had been available, but we certainly left school with a little understanding of some of the Old and New Testaments and some words of Biblical wisdom available to us in our adult lives.

We had occasional Art lessons in the one large, well-lit Art Room our School possessed. Lack of paper, paint, and other art materials, and the availability of only one Art teacher for the whole School meant that our Art lessons never seemed to last long enough, occur frequently enough, or provide enough stimulation or interest for me to become really involved in a piece of work. Our attempts at creativity were cramped and any latent talent we may have had was restricted for various reasons, mostly associated with the War. We had lost interest in whatever we had started (and often could not find our piece of work) by the time we had our next lesson.

I remember only one assignment that gave me satisfaction. We were asked to produce a Jacobean design, and I thought I had painted my various fanciful flowers and leaves with swirling stems and intricately designed patterns quite well. Some years later I designed and embroidered a fire screen with a Jacobean design as a present for my father, so perhaps some creativity and slight practical result was indirectly derived from one of my Art lessons. Apart from my Jacobean painting, my Art lessons in both Junior and Senior

School made little impression on me or developed any latent talent I might have possessed.

Needlework was my least favourite subject. My left-handedness meant that I never seemed to know which end of a seam I should work from. I am sure I was expected to sew in the same way as right-handed girls but it didn't come naturally to me and no concessions were made for 'cack-handed' left-handers. Our housekeeper was a good dressmaker and easily 'ran up' a dress on her own sewing machine, but she didn't pass on her skills to me. I never used her machine and only became familiar with my mother's old treadle sewing machine (which still stood in the corner of our drawing room) after I had left school, and necessity proved to be a suitable incentive.

In our sewing lessons we were taught how to fold, pin and tack a hem, how to do French seams and other types of seams and hand stitching. We learned to thread and use the classroom sewing machines, but so much time was wasted as we waited for our turn at one of the few machines. It required more than an afternoon's lesson for the teacher to get around the whole class to check our work. Mine often had to be unpicked. My sewing never seemed right, the hemstitches were too large, or uneven, or the machining was cockled. These lessons were a nightmare to me - apart from the opportunity for whispered conversation with friends as we waited for a turn at a sewing machine. I can only remember completing one garment; struggling over a hideous, pink flannelette nightdress, having to undo my machine stitching at one stage because I had fitted the sleeves into the armholes the wrong way round. I am sure I never wore the nightdress and don't think I even took it home.

We learned nothing about design or different kinds of fabric and there was no opportunity or encouragement for any creativity in our work. As a result of my poor achievement in needlework lessons I never became proficient at dressmaking. I am not much better at alterations and avoid having to use my sewing machine or the contents of my sewing box whenever possible. I have enjoyed doing many forms of embroidery and needlepoint in adult life, but this area of needlework was never developed at school after our initial attempts at simple embroidery stitches on Binca and felt in Infant and Junior School. Embroidery has given me much more pleasure than 'sewing' ever did.

Science should have been part of our wider curriculum at Senior School, but our Science Lab. had benches, stools and sinks, but empty cupboards. Bunsen burners were fixed to the benches but they were not used and we had no real Science lessons. We didn't learn anything at all about chemistry, physics or even human biology. We had occasional lessons in the Science Lab. but these were mainly to do with simple biology and could easily have been called 'Nature Study'. They were a little more advanced than the 'nature table' we used to have at Junior School. Our lack of Science education meant that a whole area of our lives was undeveloped.

Our P.E., gym and games lessons were high spots in my week and were a great improvement on our Junior School team games and physical jerks. The weekly P.E. lesson took place in the playground and consisted of what in my present 50+ Keep Fit Class is called 'Stretch and Tone' activity, (but without our lively music) and we older ladies have much more variety in our movement and do a lot of floor work indoors on our mats that was impossible in the playground when I was young. We used to stand in four lines, wearing our different coloured House bands, and after various warm -up exercises we played a variety of team games in the fresh air.

The School had a modern, well-equipped Gymnasium that was a distinct improvement on the hoops and balancing forms in the small school Hall of my Junior School. There were showers in the changing rooms, which were appreciated by some and disliked by others. Shy girls disliked being half undressed with their underwear exposed to all eyes, but there was no uniform P.E. kit, no shorts or special tops, and T-shirts had not been thought of. We took off our gymslips, (why were they called 'gymslips', I wonder, if we removed them for gym? - an anachronism of far earlier years of girls' education, no doubt) ties and blouses, and replaced our lace-up shoes with black plimsolls. We were left wearing our white vests tucked into the elastic at the waist of our navy blue, rather baggy, school knickers for our gym lesson, trusting that the elastic had not lost its grip.

I was not a particularly strong or muscular girl and had some difficulty in climbing up the ropes, but I found it a challenge and struggled hard to reach the top. Working with the other apparatus was somewhat easier, winding my way through the window ladder and using the ribs, box, horse and balancing on the bars. The highlight was the end of term game of 'Pirates' when every piece of equipment was set out, raffia mats were placed on any large spaces around the floor and all the apparatus was accessible. One House team was elected to chase the rest of the class and nobody was allowed to step on to the floor. If you did, you were 'out'. If the chasing team touched you, you were also 'out'. We all had to move fast and so it was quite dangerous, as the need for safe, careful footwork could easily be ignored in the enthusiasm of the chase, but our P.E. teacher was a very strict umpire, kept a close eye on her class of forty-six-or-so girls and the game made a noisy and exhilarating end to each term.

After our gym lessons we giggled and wriggled as we scampered into the showers and were hustled out again just as smartly by our gym mistress. No chance of dawdling or wasting time, just a very quick sprinkle of - hopefully - warm water, a rapid rub down with a towel and on with our uniform, before the orderly crocodile of silent girls trailed along the empty corridors of the boys' end of the school back to our own territory.

The third physical activity each week was our games period. The Council commandeered our School field during the War for use by local allotment holders, so our games were confined to the playground, where we played netball in the winter and rounders in the summer. I loved both games and in my final year I was in the School netball and rounders teams for our inter-House matches and also in the very few inter-school matches we were able to play.

The only 'away' match I remember occurred shortly before I left school in 1945, when the rounders team had the new experience of travelling by coach to a school in another district. After the match was over we sat around tables in the school dining hall and made attempts at conversation with our erstwhile opponents as we shared some simple refreshments. As I look back to those times I realise that even the development of our social skills was restricted because of the War. Inter-school matches were one of the few small changes that began to occur in the last few weeks before I left School. Other extra-curricular activities gradually appeared in the years after the War, but it was not until 1949 that the minimum school leaving age was raised to fifteen. The l944 Education Act was implemented all too slowly and far too late for me.

Our Music lessons still consisted mainly of singing. I don't recall listening to any classical records while at School, but can remember our Music teacher playing part of Beethoven's 5th Symphony as she sat at the grand piano on the stage. She told us that the BBC broadcasts to occupied Europe were always introduced by the dot-dot-dot-dash of the Morse code 'V' sign. This became known as the 'V' for Victory signal. Miss Hyde demonstrated to us that the rhythm of the well-known motif from Beethoven's 5th Symphony was identical in rhythm to the Morse code sign, telling us that this musical phrase introduced the BBC broadcasts. I don't think we learned anything about musical notation or theory (although I already read music written for the keyboard because of my piano lessons), but I may have forgotten this part of our Music syllabus.

However, our singing lessons are not forgotten, despite - or perhaps because of - the fact that our teacher was a somewhat formidable lady. We learned some lovely songs, including the words that were written to Schubert's Quintet 'The Trout' that begin with the words, 'I stood beside a brooklet that sparkled on its way.' My ex-classmate who emigrated to Australia soon after she left School can still remember the words (in English, of course; we knew no German) of all three verses of 'The Trout'. We also learned Schubert's song, 'Hark, hark, the lark, at heaven's gate sings, as Phoebus 'gins arise', although we had no idea who Phoebus was, what 'gins arise' meant, or that the words of the song had been written by Shakespeare. We were only given the words of our songs and were expected to learn them by heart.

Hymn Practice was an unmissable lesson, taking place in the School Hall immediately after Wednesday morning Assembly. John Bunyan's hymn, 'He who would valiant be' and especially, 'Immortal, invisible, God only wise' remain in my memory. Miss Hyde's insistence that we did not slide up the last syllable of 'in-vis-i-ble' has never been forgotten! She stressed, with much weight of her strong personality that we were not to give two notes to the last syllable of this word; it had *one note to each syllable* and woe betide anyone who slipped in an extra semi-quaver.

At our Remembrance Day Assembly each November we sang 'O valiant hearts, who to your glory came; through dust of conflict and through battle flame'. We were in the midst of another conflict and many of the girls had fathers away in the Armed Forces. It must have been hard for them to sing this hymn. I do not recall anyone talking about their absent fathers or discussing their personal lives at all. I was never told whether anyone knew, not even Miss Pike or my Form Mistresses, that my mother was a long-term patient in a Mental Hospital. There was never any reference to it and I kept my mouth shut on the subject. I think my friends knew that I did not have a mother at home and that a housekeeper cared for our family, even if they didn't know why, or what her status was in the household. I knew nothing about any of my classmate's family circumstances and only discovered in recent years that the father of one girl in my class had died when she was young. I have no idea how many of my classmates' fathers were in the Forces.

We had annual examinations during the Easter Term and received one Report a year at the end of this term. We were tested each year in Arithmetic, Science, History, Geography and various aspect of English: Grammar: Spelling, Dictation, Creative Writing (but still called Composition), Handwriting and our Reading ability and style, but not in Literature. What a limited range of subjects when compared with today!

Although the size of these Reports had more than doubled when compared with the tiny Reports from my Junior School, it is obvious as I read through them now and consider my education from a great distance in time, that we had a very inadequate curriculum. We learned no foreign language. Although French is printed on my Report form, it was deleted from the list of subjects we actually studied. I have an examination mark and a teacher's comment on my so-called Science lessons, but I don't think we ever lit a Bunsen burner. When we occasionally sat on the high stools in the Lab, we drew pictures or diagrams of specimens of leaf varieties, or flowers' stamens, pistils, stigmas and calyxes, propping up our elbows on the polished wooden bench-tops as we listened to our Science teacher. Wartime conditions, together with lack of essential equipment and possibly specialist teaching staff, must have been the cause of these deficiencies. The printed Reports for this six-year-old School implied that these subjects would have been taught if the world had been at peace.

Our form teachers took us for our English lessons and further encouraged my love of poetry by introducing us to many poems. We learned Tennyson's epic poem 'The Lady of Shallot' by heart. I loved the mental pictures the poem presented as the sad story unfolded, and I can still recite some of it. (Another old school friend tells me that we had to learn this poem as a punishment because nobody would own up to throwing a stone at a girl in the playground!) We memorised 'The Highwayman' by Alfred Noyes, and studied, or at least read the lengthy poem, 'The Rime of the Ancient Mariner' by Samuel Taylor Coleridge. We learned some of this strange epic; the picture of the Ancient Mariner with his 'long grey beard and glittering eye', and the haunting lines: 'Water, water everywhere, and all the boards did shrink, Water, water everywhere and not a drop to drink' have remained with me all my life. We also studied Longfellow's 'Hiawatha', and Mrs. Humphries gave me the nickname of 'Laughing Water', apparently because I was nearly always laughing - perhaps I could also have been called 'Babbling Brook' because I chattered a lot too!

Miss Pike took occasional English lessons with our class. She was very particular about our correct use of English and accurate spelling, and if she met a girl in the corridor she was likely to speak to her by name, then ask her to spell 'necessary' or 'accommodate', or whatever was the current special word. These two words particularly stick in my mind, as the entire school sometimes rhythmically recited these and other tricky words, in our morning Assembly, and I think all old Chandosians know how to spell 'ne-ce-ss-ar-y' and 'acc-omm-od-ate-' correctly. Correct speech, spelling, punctuation and grammar were considered very important. We were given a list of twenty words to learn each week at home, followed by a spelling test every Friday. I remember Miss Pike speaking to me one day in a corridor and I made some mistake in the grammatical construction of my reply. She quietly told me that I had 'split an infinitive'. At the time I was not sure what an infinitive was, but one endeavoured to please and I worked out for myself what she meant.

What a lot of time we spent learning poems, songs and parts of the Bible from memory. It may appear to be a waste of time nowadays, but portions of these poems, songs and excerpts from the Bible are still indelibly imprinted on my mind and have been a source of great pleasure over the years. If I had not learned them then, I would not have had the continued delight of the remembered lines now. There is a value in memorising, which not only develops an appreciation of words and provides a reminder of moral values, but is also an excellent exercise for the mind. Sadly in today's rush and hurry and complex curriculum there is no time. I am reminded of Kipling's poem - 'What is this life, if full of care, we have no time to stand and stare?' - it could be reworded, "What is this life, if full of IT, we have no time to sit and learn poetry?"

Our Maths teaching was rather elementary but thorough as far as it went. We had little development in our understanding of algebra or geometry, but still had plenty of mental and mechanical arithmetic lessons. We did very little practical Maths at all, although I do have a very vague recollection of leaving the classroom on one occasion with simple hand-made equipment to measure the height of some trees in the park. Our form teacher taught us Mathematics (which was simply referred to as Arithmetic on our Reports) during each of our three years at Senior School, I appear to have made good progress, gaining 80% in Arithmetic at the end of my First Year and 96% in my last year in 1945. (I can scarcely believe my eyes as I look at this result and compare it with 'Fairly Good' for Arithmetic in my last year at Priestmead School.)

One other activity was incorporated into our timetable for a short while. We had a few Dancing lessons in the School Hall. Half the girls in the class had to be the 'boys' in our Country Dancing lessons and we learned the steps and movements of a few simple folk dances. Some of my partners had clammy hands, but one poor girl suffered from eczema and had very rough, hard skin on her hands. I disliked having to hold her hand in our dances, but didn't realise then what discomfort she might be enduring. I didn't enjoy these dances; they didn't seem to go with much of a swing and were nothing like the intricate dances I do nowadays in my Folk Dance Club, despite the fact that we are all rather elderly.

An American teacher was in the School for a term and she endeavoured to teach Classic Greek Dancing to her ungainly pupils. We were not very responsive or supple in our movements and I fear that neither she, nor the class, enjoyed these occasional efforts to make us ladylike and graceful. I doubt whether many girls were able to have ballet lessons in those days. I had never heard of ballet in my childhood and certainly didn't know of any ballet classes for aspiring young dancers. Maybe Greek Dancing was a small step down the path of learning to dance, but it was a very brief introduction into the art of being graceful.

Miss Oyston taught us Geography in each of the three years I spent at Chandos School. We studied the different climatic regions of the world in our First Year - the Temperate Region, the Equatorial Region, etc. We drew graphs showing the average monthly rainfall and temperature variation, crops grown and exports (which were probably much reduced and very hazardous to transport in wartime). These areas seemed so remote and unreal in those days before the impact of televised film and news coverage came into our homes, or interviews with authentic people from 'real' countries were seen and heard. We knew of nobody who had been to these countries; we had never seen TV holiday programmes, wildlife films, or documentaries of disasters. We had never been on a school day trip, let alone a school study holiday away from home and none of us had been abroad for a holiday with our families. We didn't have multi-racial classes and knew little or nothing about other nationalities. We were the last pre-television generation to grow up or be educated in such an insular environment.

I worked hard in Miss Oyston's Geography class, drew my maps and graphs, pasted them into my exercise book and tried to make everything good enough to gain some House Marks. This seemed of more importance than gaining knowledge! My School Reports implied that I had succeeded in pleasing my teacher. Her comments 'Her work is intelligent', 'An excellent result', 'She has done well' seem to indicate that I had put my best into the subject, but I am not sure whether my understanding of the world was deepened in any way by my Geography lessons. The world 'out there' seemed very remote. Perhaps the very lack of depth and understanding in our wartime education made me thirsty for knowledge as I grew older.

Our Second Year class was even larger than the First Year. My Easter report in 1944 states that there were now forty-eight girls in the class. Our Form Mistress, Mrs. Humphries, was another good teacher, with a gentler, less robust style than Miss Oyston but who nevertheless had no difficulty in keeping nearly fifty just-teenage (we had never heard of this word!) girls in order. She taught us English and Maths in our Second Year; she also took us for History throughout my time at School. We learned some aspects of political history in the seventeenth century, with the Stuart accession - 'In 1603 James the VI of Scotland became James I of England' and events such as the Gunpowder Plot, the Plague in 1665 and the Great Fire of London in 1666. I vaguely remember having a lesson concerning Gen. Wolfe capturing the Heights of Abraham in Quebec – but didn't really appreciate where Canada was. Similarly, being told about the Boston Tea Party, but not understanding its significance, and can only remember it because of its 'oddness'. It was years before I appreciated that it concerned the revolt against the tea tax that led to the beginning of the American War of Independence. I seem to have a blank in my mind about any eighteenth century English history. We learned about the nineteenth century Industrial Revolution in our Third Year social history lessons. I remember hearing about the Luddite rebellion, the changes in agriculture with the development of agricultural equipment, the role of the inventors in the evolution of factories and large mills, and of the building of the Canals. We never caught up with the twentieth century, learned nothing about the Great War, but were, without realising it, living through one of the most historic epochs of the century.

Certainly, life would never be the same again and education would be completely altered within a few years. The limitations and restrictions we experienced would soon change when modern educational theories began to be introduced and 'Senior' School would soon be an obsolete term. It was altered to 'Secondary Modern' for some years and then, in the late l960s, the 'Comprehensive' system came into being. Not everything was ideal in my schooldays, but I look back with gratitude to the values and good basic teaching I received, whilst having a degree of envy for the educational opportunities offered to the present generation. Nevertheless there was an indefinable quality about my limited education.

Chapter Seventeen

AN UNEXPECTED HOLIDAY

Not everybody had an annual paid holiday in the 1920s and 30s, and many people only had the annual Bank Holidays at Easter, Whitsun, August and Christmas, but my father had enjoyed a week's holiday in the years prior to the War. My last family holiday with both my parents had been in Suffolk in 1938. Holidays away from home were very rare during the War years, but, although it was very difficult to get staff, Meakers had decided to give their employees a week's holiday in 1944. Four days could be taken in one week and two days in another, to ensure that there would be a full complement of staff in the shops on the busier Saturdays. This was the first holiday the staff had since 1939; maybe the management felt that the War was dragging on so long, and provided the holiday to improve morale.

My father thought that we could have a four-day cycling holiday during the School Spring half-term week, and planned to start our short break on the Sunday, using only two days of his official 'allowance' after the Bank Holiday Monday. He was due back in the shop on the Thursday. He was concerned about taking too much time off, as he felt he did not have enough responsible staff to leave in the shop in his absence. He hoped it would be possible to take the longer period of leave in the summer.

My father was accustomed to cycling eight miles every day to work and another eight miles home in the evening and I was by then quite a proficient cyclist. He joinded the Cyclists' Touring Club, and, equipped with their small booklet of accommodation addresses, we set off to Berkshire on a sunny Bank Holiday Sunday morning, with a cloudless blue sky above us. The sun had certainly 'got his hat on', and I don't think I had to have a second 'wake-up' call from my father on that day! We intended spending our brief holiday in one of the villages by the River Thames. It was going to be a very different holiday from when he had driven to Gorleston in 1938 in his Ford Eight car, with my mother at his side and me in the back. My father's thoughts - but not mine - must have gone back to that time. I had no thoughts of the past and was just anticipating our adventure together.

Our night attire, a change of clothing, toilet things and Library books (which we were hoping to read as we lazed away in the sunshine on the river-bank) were packed away into our saddle-bags, along with a brown paper bag of sandwiches for our lunch. Our waterproof capes were strapped to our cycle frames, in case the weather changed and we were caught in the rain. We must have looked very formal as we left home, with my father wearing a shirt and tie beneath his old sports jacket, his thin legs accentuated by the cycle clips round the bottom of his grey flannel trousers, while I was wearing my school blazer over a summer dress. No shorts or trousers in those days - schoolgirls didn't wear trousers!

We set off on this fine sunny morning, pedalling energetically along the traffic-free main roads. As we approached the industrial town of Slough towards mid-day, the sun grew stronger and my legs were getting tired. We cycled along the quiet, main road on the outskirts of the town and were relieved to notice a gap in the ribbon development of small houses on both sides of the road. There was a hedge on the left with a line of trees and a field beyond - a little piece of farmland that had not then been 'in filled' with housing. We were glad to have found somewhere to rest for a while. We laid our bikes on the rough grass verge beside the road – no padlocks necessary! - scrambled through an opening in the prickly hawthorn hedge, and sat in the blazing sun on the edge of the young growing wheat to eat our sandwiches. The mid-day sun was beating down on us and we soon had to move into the shade of some old trees, to cool down on the rough grass beneath, before continuing our journey. Our exertions had been fairly strenuous, and despite the use of my three-speed gears to aid me up the long hilly stretches on the open road, I felt quite worn out.

So off we set off again and eventually reached one of the villages near the River Thames. It had been a long ride and we were so glad to be at the end of our journey - or so we thought. My father produced his little handbook, checked on the list of local accommodation, and knocked at the doors of several of the recommended addresses, but none of these country cottage boarding houses could take us in. We cycled on to another village, but found that nobody had a vacancy for two weary cyclists, even though the sun was setting and the day was drawing to a close. Perhaps the requirement for two single bedrooms proved a problem in these homes - and it *was* a Bank Holiday!

It slowly dawned on me that we were far from home and had nowhere to spend the night. We had had nothing to eat since midday, but the streets seemed empty on the Bank Holiday Sunday evening, no shops were open, no restaurants or cafes could be seen. We cycled into Reading but the old county town was also deserted. We felt very downcast as we found our way to the Police Station to ask for help. I had never been near a Police Station before and was a little nervous about going in. My father asked the Constable behind the desk if he could suggest somewhere for us to stay, but he could not assist us and was not interested. We would happily have spent the night in one of the cells! It was too late, too great a distance to consider cycling all the way back home and we were certainly too tired. There was no alternative but to find the railway station and hope for a London-bound train to take us nearer to home, and the police officer gave us the directions to the Station. I am sure he was only too glad to get us out of the way.

Reading was on the main Great Western Railway line that went through Ealing Broadway Station and terminated at Paddington and we were relieved to discover that the next train stopped at Ealing Broadway Station. My father cycled to Ealing every day and knew that we would be within cycling distance of home, so able to have somewhere to sleep that night. The platform was deserted and we sat in the waiting room for some time before the train steamed in. We put our bikes in the luggage van and collapsed into our seats in an almost empty train, knowing that it would take us nearer home. When it stopped at Ealing Station we still had to cycle another eight miles before we

were back in our own home and were able to sink thankfully into our own beds. We were hungry and weary, but too tired to bother to prepare anything to eat that night. It had been an exhausting, frustrating, disappointing day.

When my father had joined the Cyclists Touring Club he had assumed that cyclists *toured*, that it wasn't necessary to pre-book, and had not considered it necessary to reserve our accommodation in advance, but we discovered that this assumption was incorrect. In normal circumstances it probably wasn't necessary, but our requirements were not normal; we were away on a Bank Holiday Weekend and also required accommodation in two bedrooms, which these small country cottages might not have had.

The following day he went to our local public phone box near our parade of shops and made a number of calls, trying to book accommodation nearer the end of my half term holiday. (One wouldn't dream of taking a holiday in term time.) At last he was successful; two rooms were available in the latter part of the week in a cottage in the small village of Sonning near to the river. He made a provisional booking for three nights from the Thursday to the Saturday night, but he then had to get permission to have the Saturday off work. In view of the circumstances his employer gave consent and he was able to confirm our booking. We began our holiday on the Thursday, and, instead of getting back to work for the busy Saturday's trade, we were able to come home on the Sunday in time for Monday morning and school.

So we returned to the Berkshire countryside a day or two later. This time we cycled from Kenton to Kingsbury, along the Edgware Road and on to Paddington Station. After putting our cycles in the luggage van, we travelled with more ease and much more speed on a fast train to Reading. We steamed through Ealing Station and remembered how tired we had been there a few days before. We alighted at Reading, retrieved our bikes and began our cycle ride to Sonning. It had been a much more enjoyable start to the holiday. My father had not appreciated that miles pedalled on a bicycle seem much longer than the miles he had driven in his car on the pre-War excursions to the Thames-side beauty spots with my mother! The previous long cycle ride from home to our destination had been a waste of a day's holiday.

The weather was still fine and sunny, and the wild roses and early honeysuckle were blooming in the hedgerows. In his desire to produce a happy atmosphere and in his pleasure at having succeeded at last in getting away on holiday, my father began to sing one of his old songs, 'You are my honey, honeysuckle, I am the bee' as we cycled along the country lanes. (No doubt he had sung this song years ago, around the piano with my mother and his sister- and brother-in-law.) At last our holiday had actually begun and he was feeling very pleased and light-hearted. His anxieties and burdens were lifted for a while.

I recall nothing about the house we stayed in, but I do recollect cycling along the quiet country lanes, joining in with my father in his 'Honeysuckle' song and sitting in the bright spring sunshine by the riverside reading my Library book. But one afternoon the sun was too strong to read; my eyelids drooped and I nodded off to sleep. We had been reading and enjoying the fine weather and had both dozed off in a field by the riverbank. I was suddenly awakened by a snuffling sound. I slowly opened my eyes and looked up to make the alarming discovery that a cow was peering down at me, its head uncomfortably close to mine, and its' legs mingling with my bike that was lying on the grass beside me. My father heard my cry of shock and awoke with a start, and we realised that our quiet little spot had been invaded by a herd of cows. No doubt they felt that we had encroached upon their territory, and with thumping hearts we beat a hasty retreat.

I met a similar herd of cows when on a Thames-side towpath walk not so long ago. They were chomping the lush grass by the side of the river; they ignored my husband and I, stood right in our path, and *we* had to get out of *their* way. It brought back vivid memories of the incident of so long ago. The cows still thought it was their preserve and still made no concessions to ramblers on the towpath.

Our brief holiday passed all too quickly, the weather had changed, and on the Sunday morning we packed our belongings into our saddlebags and began the journey home. We cycled along the narrow peaceful lanes once more until we reached the outskirts of Reading and then stopped on the Bridge to have a last look at the river before pedalling on to the Station. As we looked up-river we were amazed to see a continuous line of boats moored alongside the riverbank. We walked across to the other side of the road and looked down-river, and there we saw another armada of boats. They had suddenly appeared overnight. We had been near the river for a few days and had noticed no unusual signs of marine activity, but it was obvious that there had been a huge movement of landing craft during the night. All the boats were facing downstream, but there was not a soul in sight or a sound to be heard. It was a memorable, but quite eerie, and certainly a breath-taking, sight. My father commented thoughtfully that he was sure 'something big' was about to happen. I was baffled at the sight of so many boats and couldn't understand where they could have come from so suddenly.

After watching the scene for some while, pondering over its significance, we cycled on to the station and caught our train. On arrival at Paddington, we retrieved our bicycles from the luggage van, left the Station and cycled into Praed Street before turning into the Edgware Road, the A5, as I now know it. We had quite a long cycle ride along an empty Edgware Road before turning left into the Kingsbury Road and on to the familiar streets of Kenton. If I had known what would be required of me at the end of that eventful year I would have taken a lot more notice of the details of my immediate surroundings when we got off the train, and the route we took, but my father and I had little foreknowledge of coming events, although he had correctly anticipated the major event that occurred early the following week.

What we had gazed at on the bridge over the River Thames that Sunday morning was some of the preparation for the imminent invasion of Europe. Two days later on Tuesday, June 6th, we learned from the news bulletin on the wireless that the long-anticipated invasion had begun; D-Day had arrived. My father's comment of 'something big about to happen' has been remembered, together with the mental picture of the lines of boats we had seen two days previously. The few vivid memories of honeysuckle, rose hedges, cows and armada of small boats moored at the river's edge have blanked out any other recollections of this brief holiday. We had had a tiny glimpse of the preparations for the Allied Invasion of Europe and seen some of the landing craft on their way to the Normandy beaches. Throughout the coming weeks everybody listened intently to the news on the Home Service of the fighting across the Channel, and followed the gradual progress of the Allied Forces as they fought their way across Europe, liberating the people from Nazi domination as they went.

A week after D-Day, Germany retaliated by attacking the South East of England with pilotless aircraft, which were given various names - 'doodlebugs' 'buzz bombs' and 'flying bombs'. They were indeed 'flying bombs' and their official name was V1s. The noisy engines of these pilotless bombs had a rasping, throbbing sound that was accompanied by heavy vibration, which combined to make them sound very frightening. One listened intently to the noise in the air as the ghastly machine approached. When the engine suddenly cut out, there were a few seconds of ominous silence before the device plummeted to the ground, followed by a terrifying explosion. This silence was unforgettably menacing to all who heard it. This further air bombardment totally disrupted our daily life, our sleep and our education yet again. These 'doodlebugs' appeared at any time of the day or night, sometimes without any prior air raid warning, as they were launched haphazardly from across the Channel. They were not directed at any particular target, but their purpose was solely to terrify and demoralise the civilian population in the southeast of England. Some of the raids continued for so long that we did not know if the 'All Clear' had sounded during the early hours of the morning and we had slept through it. I sometimes went to off to school while an air raid was still in progress, and was directed immediately into the shelters on arrival at school.

Although these air raids sometimes lasted for hours, there was often no immediate threat, no activity, and only ominous silence for long periods, until the noise of an occasional flying bomb was heard in the distance. The noise rapidly increased as it flew into the vicinity, sometimes followed by the eventual sudden explosion. At other times the buzz bomb rumbled on overhead, passed us before the engine cut out, and exploded elsewhere. It was an eerie, nerve-racking time. I remember no sound of anti-aircraft guns, or fighter aeroplanes; there was only the occasional sickening throb from the engine of one of these missiles as it came nearer and the noise grew louder. There was a famous cartoon at that time depicting a crowd of people in a street, each with a huge right ear, listening intently for a flying bomb.

Again we were forced to spend the best part of many summer days sitting in very dim light on the backless wooden benches of the school air raid shelters. The sun was shining outside but once again we had to occupy ourselves with our pencil and paper games in the gloomy underground. It was impossible for the staff to do any proper teaching, as their voices did not carry clearly through the long tunnel of the dugout shelter. There was no space in which to move around; we could not hear the day-to-day sounds of the wind and the birds in the outside world, nor see daylight, blue sky and summer sunshine. It was certainly not a place for anyone who suffered from claustrophobia.

At last the single-toned note of the 'All Clear' sounded and we were released into the playground for fifteen minutes of fresh air and exercise to 'let off steam'. No doubt our teachers hoped to enjoy a short break, a cup of tea in the Staff Room, and the opportunity for some brief relaxation before returning to their classrooms. However, during those last weeks of the summer term, the whine of the air raid warning often sounded once again before we had even had time to settle down to a lesson. Back to the shelters we scuttled. I don't remember any bad behaviour or lack of co-operation from any of my schoolmates during those days. We were all fed up with the life we had to lead, frightened by the bombing and probably tired through lack of sleep. Our teachers had a stressful time too, with a tunnel full of youngsters cooped up for hours, with loads of bottled-up energy, together with their concerns that the syllabus was not being completed, and their pupils' education and future prospects were being jeopardised.

My father, our housekeeper and Rose had all gone to work one morning during this period. I was at the sink washing up the breakfast dishes before setting off for school when I noticed the irregular drone of a doodlebug engine throbbing in the distance and knew that something nasty was rapidly getting louder and nearer. Our larder was built under the staircase; we stored our potatoes and kept the shopping basket beneath the deep tiled shelf that went from the back of the larder almost to the door. The space under the shelf was too small for all the family to take shelter in but I had been told to use it in an emergency if I was alone in the house. As the 'buzz bomb' drew nearer and the noise increased, my fear increased too and I ran to the larder, bobbed down into my safe place, pulling the larder door almost – but not quite - closed.

The drone of the flying bomb grew ever closer and I crouched low in this dark cramped space beside the basket of King Edward potatoes. I waited, heart in my mouth, hoping that the engine would not cut out, but fearing that the bomb was about to drop. As the engine sound increased I grew really scared, until it suddenly stopped and all was quiet for a few moments, with a silence that could almost be felt. Then there was a tremendous crash. I had no idea where the bomb had fallen. It had seemed so near, but there was no sound of falling debris, so I knew that our house was safe.

When I emerged from my little refuge I discovered that the surrounding houses were still standing and the flying bomb had fallen some distance away. It had seemed overhead to my ears, but it had not flown right over our house and had exploded before it reached my road. My first thought was for my father. I knew he was cycling to work in the same direction that the noise of the flying bomb had appeared to be coming from. I learned later that after the explosion he had turned around and cycled back towards home to see if I was all right. He came near to the area where the bomb had fallen and was not allowed to pass through, but from that he knew that I was not involved, as the site of the explosion was not in the immediate vicinity of our home. The bomb had dropped midway between us. I had no such assurance about my father's safety until he came home from work that evening, and I saw that he was alive and well. When I had realised in the morning that I was in no immediate danger I had dashed off to school, and was sent straight to the shelters. Such was life in those days. Oh, for a mobile phone then!

The return of nightly air raids had made my father consider the necessity of sleeping in the air raid shelter again, but our Anderson shelter in the garden was now uninhabitable. The raids were so frightening and dangerous that he decided we should make use of the street shelters at bedtime. We were joined by some of our neighbours who were of the same mind. These public, brick, aboveground shelters (fun to bounce balls against, but not pleasant to sleep in) were built at the sides of many minor roads. We took our bedclothes with us each evening; each family chose a separate part of the shelter and we spread out our blankets and pillows on the hard, slatted, wooden bunks and tried to get to sleep. There was no privacy and it was very uncomfortable. One of our neighbours snored very heavily and the sound seemed to reverberate around the brick walls of the shelter, so we had little sleep. It was almost (but not quite) like the sound of an approaching doodlebug!

We were also disturbed during the night by what we thought was the sound of a hedgehog that had made its home somewhere in the shelter and resented our intrusion - like the cows by the side of the river! In spite of our nightly searches with the aid of a torch and a stick, we could not locate or remove it. We only spent a few nights there before abandoning the street shelter, just as we had forsaken our garden Anderson shelter during the Blitz. We went back to our own beds. The continual discomforts and irritations of communal sleeping and the small permanent resident of the shelter appeared greater than the intermittent fear of the sound of an occasional doodlebug or of being victims of a direct hit. The hedgehog kept its territory and we returned to our own home.

As the summer term went on it became evident that there were fewer and fewer girls in my once large class of forty-eight pupils. I don't think I understood that many had already been evacuated, or had moved away to stay with relatives or friends who lived in other, safer, parts of the country, far away from the danger zone in the southeast. Our end of year Assembly had been a very special occasion in our large School Hall at the end of my First Year, but this year the Education Authority had decreed that it was too dangerous to have the whole school in one place indoors. It would take too long to empty the School Hall and get everyone into the shelters quickly if there was an air raid. Chairs were brought out into the playground and placed in rows near the shelters for our final Assembly and a much depleted school group sat in the open air on the last afternoon of the Summer Term. Missing from this Assembly was the stage; there was no piano in the playground for Miss Hyde to accompany our singing of the School Hymn. Miss Pike addressed us from behind a small table on which was displayed the School Shield as usual, ready to have the new House winner's coloured ribbon tied around it, but the usual atmosphere of our Assemblies had gone.

I remember that Assembly very clearly, not only because it was held in the playground, but also because it was the occasion on which I was awarded a 'posture badge'. Posture badges were presented at the end of each term to the girls who had been observed by members of Staff to be sitting up straight in class, who walked about the school with their heads up, shoulders back and who did not slouch at their desks. When my name was called I walked across the playground, and Miss Pike came from behind the small table to present me with my badge. The small brooch, covered with material in the School colours was pinned to my gymslip. I was pleased and proud to receive it, but somehow it seemed less important in the informal outdoor surroundings, with so few to share my brief moment of glory. No appointments of Head Girl or Prefects for the coming School Year were announced. The future was unknown at that time and there were so few girls still at School.

Miss Pike did announce the name of the winning House for the current School Year, but enthusiasm was diminished and the atmosphere in the playground was rather tense, with the nearby shelters almost beckoning us back into their gloomy tunnels. We sang the School Hymn at the close of our Assembly, but the sound was very feeble in the open air with so few present and without Miss Hyde's usual rousing piano accompaniment, it dissipated in the gentle breeze of that sunny afternoon. The usual fervour of our end of term Assemblies was absent on this very low-key occasion.

The doodlebugs had blighted the last part of my second year at Chandos. The summer holidays began with the prospect of more air raids and without much to look forward to in the coming weeks… or so I thought.

Chapter Eighteen

SAFETY IN SOMERSET

The flying bomb attacks showed no sign of slackening and during the summer term the local education authority had offered evacuation to safer areas for those still at school. I wasn't aware of this official proposal at the time, and knew nothing of it until many years after the War had ended, but I had noticed that many girls had 'disappeared' from school and that our class numbers seemed to lessen with each passing day. In view of all the changes of home I had had before the War, my father may have been reluctant to send me away to an unknown family, and I have to presume that some discussion took place between my father and our housekeeper about a temporary safe home for me.

'Auntie' had friends who lived in Somerset, but I had not been told that as soon as the school holidays began I was going to stay with the sister of these friends. Almost immediately after the end of term I was surprised to learn that 'Auntie' and I were going to have a week's holiday in the country and were travelling by train from Paddington to the West Country.

Two small cases were packed and 'Auntie' and I set off for this holiday. It was a new experience for me to have such a long journey by train to the town of Wellington, near Taunton. 'Auntie' was very pleased to see her old friends again when they met us at the station. They chatted together as we walked to her friend's sister's home, where 'Auntie' and I were introduced to the lady with whom we were going to stay. We shook hands with Miss Rowe, a grey-haired lady with an attractive, soft, West Country accent, who lived in a detached bungalow not far away from the Railway Station. I was shown to a nicely furnished bedroom and told that this would be my bedroom while I was staying in Wellington.

A day or two later Miss Rowe, 'Auntie' and I had a day at the seaside, with a train ride to Weston-super-Mare. It was a disappointing outing on a dull chilly day. The promenade was deserted; huge rolls of anti-invasion barbed wire were stretched all along the sea front, preventing us from going on to the beach. The tide was out and I couldn't even see the sea as I gazed through the mist into the far distance. We walked along the promenade on this damp, wild, blustery day, occasionally peering through the barbed wire at the empty beach, trying to catch a glimpse of the sea. I could scarcely believe that the Bristol Channel was really out there beyond the great expanse of wet sand. It was not like the summer visits to the seaside I had previously enjoyed with my parents, or at Bournemouth with my Aunt and Uncle in 1939.

We were eating our breakfast a few days later when Miss Rowe left the dining table and went into the kitchen to refill the teapot. I was eating my corn flakes, holding my spoon – as I usually did - above the handle, instead of beneath, which helped to keep my left hand steady. 'Auntie' took the opportunity to correct my table manners, telling me (once again!) how to hold the spoon in the proper way. Although it felt awkward for a long time, I never held my spoon incorrectly from that day on! That memory mingles with the information she went on to give me, explaining that I was not going back to Kenton with her at the end of the week, but was to remain with Miss Rowe until it was safer at home. The initial short stay had been arranged as a trial period to see whether this spinster lady felt able to live with the intrusion of a thirteen-year-old girl living in her home for an indefinite period. Our housekeeper also wanted to ensure that I appeared to have settled down in these new surroundings.

I was really surprised to hear this news and it was quite a shock to know that I was not going home. I had gleaned no idea of this plan and overheard no conversations concerning it. This news and the spoon incident are irrevocably entwined in my memory. 'Auntie' returned to Kenton alone at the end of the week, and I soon got used to living in another home. I learned that when the school holiday was over I would attend the local girls' Senior School where Miss Rowe was a teacher.

Miss Rowe wanted to go to Plymouth a few days later and so she and I had another day out, with another train journey. Plymouth had been very badly bombed in the Blitz and my main memory of our visit to this famous City is a mental picture of vast devastated areas, gaunt remains of dirty grey buildings, with an occasional isolated church spire or solitary building still standing. Many little shops were closed and boarded up; it appeared to be a dead City. I had not seen anything of the terrible ruins in the City of London, the Docks, or the East End, but the bomb damage in Plymouth was much worse than anything I had come across on our shopping trips to the West End of London earlier in the War.

Miss Rowe was very upset to see Plymouth looking so bomb-scarred. She was very shocked at the extent of the destruction and I had the impression that she had not been there since the heavy bombing of the City, or had not realised the extent of the devastation. She could not find the store she had wanted for her particular purchase. It had been destroyed. She appeared to be quite stunned as we made our way back to the station through the ruins and was very quiet on the journey home. It seems strange that so soon after I was evacuated I saw more signs in the West of England of the preparations for invasion and more results of the air attacks than I had seen at home throughout the War.

Apart from these gloomy reminders of the War, I was soon very happy in Wellington and enjoyed the few months I spent living in Miss Rowe's comfortable home. There were no air raids, no flying bombs, no disruption of lessons at school and no broken nights, in this small, sleepy country town. Miss Rowe and I got on well together. Her niece was in the Sixth form at a Boarding School in Bristol, and lived with her Aunt during her school holidays. Joan arrived soon after 'Auntie' returned home. Her mother was also a long-term patient in a Mental Hospital, so we should have had something in common, but neither of us ever mentioned our mothers or compared our circumstances. Were we subconsciously ashamed of the stigma of 'mental illness'? In the climate of the period, had we both been quietly encouraged to forget our mothers? In retrospect, I believe it would have been very comforting to talk to someone in circumstances somewhat similar to own. Joan was also an only child. I don't know how long her mother had been ill, or whether she remained in Hospital for the rest of her life as my mother did, and often wonder how Joan's life turned out. I have met no one else whose mother has spent most of her daughter's life as a patient in a Psychiatric Hospital. It was certainly isolating for my father and, I now realise, for me, to have nobody else with whom to share the experience of the absence of a wife or a mother due to severe mental illness. I wonder why Joan and I didn't share our experience.

Joan was able to come home for the rest of her school holiday after 'Auntie' returned to Kenton. She slept in the spare bed in her aunt's twin-bedded room when I was living in her home and I didn't understand at the time that this was because I had been given her bedroom. She was probably very annoyed that she had been deprived of her bedroom, but I didn't appreciate the disturbance I must have caused, or that she might have resented my presence as well as this temporary loss of her bedroom. I hope she was not too upset by my intrusion into her home, but with hindsight, I think she was probably furious, and we didn't seem to make any kind of friendly relationship. She was several years older than I and was a very quiet, studious girl. She always seemed to me to be very solitary and spoke very little, but maybe she was quietly showing her disapproval of my presence. I discovered nothing from her about real life at Boarding School. With my love of schoolgirl stories, which were always set in Boarding Schools, with 'dorms' and 'midnight feasts', I could have learned something about the real thing, which was possibly very different in those days from the seemingly idyllic life portrayed in fiction.

Meanwhile Miss Rowe was trying to arrange to take us both on a week's holiday, and Joan and I soon learned that we were off to a village in the Quantock Hills near Minehead for a few days. We travelled to our holiday destination by bus to Taunton, then another West Country bus to the village of

Sampford Brett near Minehead. The bus stopped on the main road near the village and we had to walk to our accommodation carrying our small suitcases. Rose Cottage had tiny rooms and no electricity. We were each given a candle every evening to show us our way to bed. When I woke in the mornings I often lay in my little bed looking at the beamed ceiling and listening to the sound of pigeons cooing - or were they doves? On hearing this sound now I am always reminded of my early morning awakening so long ago to the soft murmuring sound of these birds. I hadn't heard that sound before and was unsure at first what the strange noise could be. We didn't have pigeons, or doves, in suburban Kenton.

We explored a little of the countryside during our holiday, going for walks or taking bus rides to Blue Anchor Bay, Minehead and Dunster. One day we went to Watchet and bought some pasties from a baker's shop for our lunch. As we sat on the little beach by the harbour eating our warm pasties - filled with potato, herbs and onion - a swarm of sand flies arose from the seaweed left straggling along the shoreline by the ebb tide. These nasty little flies were so irritating and became such a nuisance that we were driven away from the beach to eat our lunch elsewhere. Nevertheless it was an enjoyable little holiday, with plenty of sunshine, and the peace and beauty of the Somerset countryside was a wonderful contrast to the frightening weeks of the flying bombs in Middlesex earlier in the summer, with their constant threat to life and home.

The school holidays came to an end. Joan returned to her Boarding School and I began the autumn term at Courtland Road School. This was the local Senior School, but it was very small compared with the large, modern one I had attended for the previous two years. There were only three classes and the school had only three teachers. The Headmistress taught the Third Year (known as the top class). Miss Yandle and Miss Rowe taught the First and Second Years (Years 7 and 8) in a large room, which was divided by folding doors across the middle, separating the two lower classes. I should have been in the Third Year (Year 9), but it was decided that I should be placed in the class of the teacher I knew. The Headmistress was rather a fearsome lady, a bit of a dragon and I think it was an 'act of mercy' to put me into Miss Rowe's class! Consequently I did not find the work very demanding. I remember little about the lessons in this School, apart from learning about the Whigs and the Tories and having a mock election in the class history lessons with Miss Yandle. I don't remember whether I voted Whig or Tory! I think we must have covered a different period in history from what had been done at Chandos. It was possibly what we should have been taught during our weeks in the shelters.

My strongest memory of that term was being taught how to weave in our craft lessons. Wellington had been famous in the past for its woollen industry, and a large family-owned woollen mill in a nearby village was probably responsible for initiating the teaching of weaving in the school. They may have been the suppliers of the wooden-framed handlooms and the various coloured skeins of wool we used. Each girl had a loom, which was small enough to be placed on the desktop during craft lessons. At the beginning of term we set up our looms with woollen thread to produce the warp, and then wound contrasting coloured wool around the shuttle before slipping it to and fro between the long threads to produce the weft.

It was very satisfying to see the cloth begin to appear as I worked at my little loom, and I found our weaving lessons with Miss Rowe much more enjoyable than my needlework lessons at Chandos. I made up my own checked patterns by choosing different colours and changing the colour of the wool in the shuttle from time to time, to design an 'original' check pattern. I was very proud of the brightly patterned scarves I wove during the term I was at Courtland Road School, and took them home in December to give as Christmas presents.

Miss Rowe and I went for a walk one Sunday afternoon to the nearby village of Tonedale where the mill was situated. It looked a large, rather grim old building that dominated the village, and at the time I didn't appreciate its industrial importance to the prosperity and employment of the nearby town. During the summer holiday period and on fine weekends we often went out for walks in the local countryside. Wellington Monument is a conspicuous landmark a few miles away on the Blackdown Hills. The obelisk commemorates the Duke of Wellington, who took his title from the town. Miss Rowe and I had a long ramble to this spot one Saturday in the autumn and had a picnic tea as we sat beneath the stone Monument, looking at the view of the green fields and hills of Somerset. We picked hazelnuts from the hedgerow as we walked home and cracked them open to eat the sweet little nuts inside while listening to the wireless in the evening. The M5 now runs across our route to the hilltop, but in the nineteen-forties we were able to walk to the Monument by quiet roads and through the fields by footpaths without having to cross this busy dual-carriage major highway.

I took part in a gymnastic display in Taunton near the end of the term, and after practising for several weeks with Miss Yandle, trying to perfect our movements, the special day arrived. First of all the coach collected the girls who lived in the town, then the driver went around the surrounding villages to pick up those who lived in outlying homes and farms, and we all drove off to Taunton. It gave me a little understanding of a very different, rural way of life from what I was used to. Some of these girls lived on farms in agricultural areas that seemed quite remote to me. I had only known of people living in terraced or detached houses in towns, or suburban streets of semi-detached houses. It was a revelation to me to find that some of the girls in my class lived in seemingly isolated houses surrounded by fields, and with no immediate neighbours.

There were no facilities for Domestic Science lessons at the school in Wellington. I had enjoyed my cookery lessons at Chandos, and Miss Rowe allowed me to experiment with some of my recipes in her kitchen. Cheese croquettes appeared quite frequently on our 'menu' for tea in the evenings! I think she was pleased to have someone who liked cooking in her home, and I was delighted to have the opportunity of using the skills I had learned, and appreciated her praise. She had a bumper crop of runner beans that summer and found various ways of making the most of them while they were tender. After our return from school I often went down the garden path to the row of beans to pick enough for our evening meal. One of her favourite dishes was to make a cheese sauce and pour it over a big plate of these freshly picked and just-cooked runner beans. She was fond of pepper and used to put plenty of pepper in her sauce. I liked this addition; it was new to me, as our housekeeper didn't use pepper in her cooking, and it made the sauce more piquant. We didn't have the variety of spices and herbs that are available today.

Miss Rowe also had some fruit trees in her garden and after picking the crop of crab apples one Saturday in early autumn we made crab-apple jelly with the pale pink-tinged fruits. Her eating apples were rather maggoty, but nevertheless we picked them all as they ripened and gathered the windfalls from the lawn as well. We sat in our easy chairs in the lounge during the evening, each with a kitchen knife, slicing through the apples and cutting out the bad bits, but eating the remaining sound parts of the fruit. The apples would not keep for long, so we ate flavoursome English Cox's apples every day for several weeks. We went black-berrying in the late summer and then made blackberry jelly, pouring the boiling sweet syrup into warmed jam pots, covering the jars with greaseproof paper and setting them on the window sill to cool and 'set'. It was very satisfying to spread the dark fruity jelly on our bread and butter for our Sunday tea. I had quite a number of new and pleasant experiences during my months living in the country; Miss Rowe and I were very companionable.

Wellington was a sleepy little town in those days. The weekly shopping was done at the local shops, and as I was used to doing a lot of the shopping back at home, I was able to help

Miss Rowe in a similar way. I set off with a purse, shopping list and basket on Saturday mornings to get the vegetables and any other items that were needed. The little shops had some of their goods displayed in wooden boxes outside. The queues were nowhere near as long as at home, but service was leisurely in the small country town and I listened to the soft Somerset accent of the local housewives as I waited my turn to be served. Everyone seemed much more relaxed and unhurried. Most of the vegetables were grown locally.

Miss Rowe wrote out a list of the groceries in an order book each week and this was handed in to the local grocer's shop on our way home from school, together with our ration cards. These were marked, coupons or 'points' cut out and the precious books were returned to us. The following Saturday morning a delivery boy appeared at the back door, with a large basket fixed on to the handlebars of his bicycle containing our groceries. The baker also called at the house in a similar way on Saturday mornings. I had not come across deliveries of food before, and it was many years before they recurred in the form of supermarket vans rushing around our roads with present-day customers' orders.

We had always carried all our shopping home in Kenton, but this delivery service made life a lot easier, especially as both Miss Rowe and I were at school all day and shops were not open at all hours at that time. We might call in at the butcher's shop on our way home in the afternoon. He made very good sausages, which I don't think were rationed and Miss Rowe sometimes bought some for our tea. We didn't eat sausages at home and I looked forward to 'sausage days'. She would order our little joint of meat for the weekend and this was also delivered on Saturday morning. I didn't know then that the butcher had been such a good friend so many years ago...

Well over fifty years later I visited the small village of Sampford Brett for the first time since 1944 and spent a night in a guesthouse a few doors away from the cottage in which I had stayed so long ago. I was reminiscing to our landlady about my evacuation to Wellington and my first visit to her village. She mentioned that there was a retired teacher living in the village who knew all the history of the area. She contacted this lady while my husband and I were out walking in the Quantock Hills during the day, and learned that she had taught at a school in Wellington during the War. By a very strange coincidence, just as we were leaving the guesthouse after breakfast the following morning, this elderly lady walked along the pavement on her way to church. Our landlady pointed her out to me and I went across and introduced myself, explaining that I had stayed in Sampford Brett in I944 and had been a pupil at Courtland Road School in Wellington. To my complete amazement she replied that she had taught at the same School during the War. I asked this lady for her name and as soon as she said it was Miss Yandle, I remembered that she had taught me history and P.E She also remembered me and recalled that I had lived with Miss Rowe.

She told me that Miss Rowe had been enquiring around the town in the summer of 1944 if anyone knew where she could take her niece and an evacuee (me!) on a holiday. It was the butcher in Wellington who gave Miss Rowe the address in Sampford Brett, where he had a relative who could - and would - accommodate us. It was an extraordinary experience to stand in a village street in I998 and talk with someone who had taught me in the school I attended for one term in I944, who had known Miss Rowe, remembered me, and was able to explain to me the origin of the holiday I was lucky enough to enjoy so long ago. The butcher certainly did us a great kindness.

I had my first introduction to freshly ground coffee while I lived in Wellington. Miss Rowe loved 'real' coffee and on our occasional bus trips into Taunton we were led unfailingly to the coffee shop by the delicious aroma wafting on the air as we approached. Miss Rowe couldn't resist the temptation to buy some of this rather expensive, freshly ground coffee. I had never smelt 'real' coffee before and the aroma of coffee grinding - rare nowadays, with most coffee pre-packed - still evokes memories of the months I spent in Somerset. Miss Rowe had an unusual way of making her coffee, sprinkling two tablespoonfuls of coffee over the top of a saucepan of milk and then heating this slowly on the gas stove. When the grains had sunk to the bottom, the coffee was carefully strained into our cups. It was an occasional special treat that we enjoyed in the evening as we sat around the sitting room fire.

She also made a kind of clotted cream, by leaving a pan of milk on top of the kitchen boiler overnight and then skimming off the thick creamy skin that had slowly formed across the top of the milk by the following morning. This was cooled and then served with some stewed fruit later in the day. We poured the rest of the skimmed milk over our corn flakes for breakfast. We appeared to have a lot more milk in the country than at Kenton and the rich milk from Somerset cows enabled Miss Rowe to make this home-produced cream from time to time, at a time when it was not available in the shops.

I wrote letters home to my father. (I am sure that Miss Rowe made certain that her 'resident pupil' kept in touch). I can recall hearing the unusual sound of my father's voice on the telephone when he rang from the shop to say that he was coming to visit me during my half-term holiday. (Although there was a telephone installed in Miss Rowe's bungalow, a long-distance 'social call' would have been considered a great extravagance in those days and it was certainly not permitted on a business line.) He still had a few days' leave due to him because of the alteration in our holiday in the spring. That enforced change of plan was going to bring us together for a little while, enabling us to have another very short holiday (and no doubt enabling Joan to enjoy sleeping in her own bedroom during her half-term break). With hindsight I wonder whether the holiday was arranged so that Joan could come home for her half-term holiday and sleep in her own bedroom!

My father travelled to Taunton Station on the Saturday overnight Royal Mail train. He told me it had stopped at every station on its journey to off-load the Mailbags. He said this procedure was very noisy and disturbing throughout the night and he had had no sleep. The remaining Mail was removed when the train arrived at Taunton in the early hours of Sunday morning, and the near empty train was then shunted into a siding. He was the only remaining passenger and he sat in an empty carriage attached to the empty train for the rest of the night. But at last it was quiet and still and he told me he lay along the seat and tried to doze for an hour or two. When the local service commenced a few hours later he was able to complete his journey to Wellington. The Royal Mail Night train stopped its service in 2004.

Miss Rowe lived close to the Station and when we heard the train hooting in the distance to announce its imminent arrival, I ran down the road to meet my father at the station. It seemed a long time since we had seen each other. He looked so tired when I saw him walking down the platform. He had been on his feet for the whole of the busy Saturday before getting on the overnight train. I am sure that the strain of the air raids of the previous months had taxed his strength and nervous energy too. I was so pleased to see him and overjoyed that not only had he arrived, but that he had brought my beloved bicycle with him too. He had cycled to Ealing on my bike on the Saturday morning and then put it in the luggage van when he got on the GWR train at Ealing Broadway Station in the evening.

I wheeled my bike along the pavement in Station Road as we walked together to the bungalow, where I introduced my father to Miss Rowe. She was a reserved lady and seemed a little shy and nervous at meeting my father. She had cooked some bacon in the oven for his breakfast, cooking it slowly; as we did not know at what time he would arrive. My father became quite ill later on in the day and he was sure that the special locally cured bacon had been insufficiently cooked and that it was the cause of his sickness! It was probably a combination of the long journey, very little sleep, the continual jolting of the train rattling over the railway lines, followed a big cooked breakfast that he was not used to. He was certainly not now accustomed to eating bacon! It made the start of our time together a little fraught.

Another brief holiday had been arranged at Rose Cottage – thanks once again to the butcher's mediation - and after a little rest (but before he became unwell) my father and I set off for Taunton, where we waited a long time for the Minehead bus. The bus conductor called out, "Move down along there" – a real Somerset phrase, as people crowded on to the bus. Journeys were very long-drawn out in those days, especially on Sundays, but eventually I arrived at Sampford Brett for a second time.

Our brief holiday in the beautiful Somerset countryside near the Quantock Hills was a very peaceful interlude for my father, away from the flying bombs and other worries at home. We went for walks, took bus rides to Minehead and other nearby places, then managed to find somewhere for a meal before we returned to the cottage each evening. We went to bed early as it soon grew dark in the autumn evenings and there was no electric light in the cottage, only gaslight in the downstairs rooms. We each had our candle to light our way up the steep, narrow, curving staircase to our bedrooms. In the morning our kind landlady brought a cup of tea and a slice of bread and thick Somerset cream to our low-ceilinged, black-beamed, white-walled bedrooms. I sat up in bed to eat this special treat, trying not to leave any crumbs or smears of cream on the white candlewick bedspread. My father was really skinny and our landlady must have thought that he needed fattening up. I don't think either of us put on any weight with our bread and cream before breakfast, but it was an unheard-of treat in our experience.

This autumn holiday was over all too soon and we had to return to Wellington on the Thursday. I waved 'goodbye' to my father at the station as he returned home. I don't remember being upset at not going home with him; I think I was enjoying my life in the country with Miss Rowe. I now had my beloved bicycle, but strangely I didn't use it very much. It was dark after we had had our tea and the damp autumn weather did not entice me out after school. The area was hilly and I didn't really know my way around to go off for rides into the country lanes. I tended to stay indoors with Miss Rowe in my free time. I think we were quite good companions in her pleasant, peaceful, comfortably furnished home and we soon had a bright fire glowing after our day at school.

I had only a little homework to do in the evenings and I didn't appear to miss my out-of-school ball games, the Library, Saturday morning cinema or playing with my friend Joan. Life had been quite weird during the weeks of flying bombs; people disappeared suddenly and I didn't know where they had gone to; we couldn't go out to play after tea; our days at school had been quite abnormal. I didn't even know that Joan had become an evacuee until many years afterwards and we didn't write to each other during these months.

The small School I attended in Wellington had four Houses named Brendon, Mendip, Quantock and Blackdown, after the surrounding ranges of hills, but there was not the keen competition between the Houses that we had at Chandos. I have no recollection of anyone being given House Marks for good work or losing House Marks for bad behaviour. There were exams and annual reports at the end of the Easter term at Chandos, but we had exams at the end of the Christmas term at Courtland Road School, followed of course by a School Report. I still have this Report and read that we were tested in Reading, English Literature (I can't remember what we studied), Composition, Spelling, Arithmetic, Recitation, Geography, History and Handwriting (my lowest mark!). We were also given a grade in Scripture, Drawing, Singing, Physical Drill, Needlework and Hygiene. This small, country School gave a Report that was much more extensive, though basic, than my large modern School at home. I think the educational and social effects of the War must have been far greater in Middlesex than in Somerset. I remember little of my lessons that term, but as I received good marks on my Report I presume I was an acceptable student. I remember even less about the girls in my class. I didn't make friends with anyone in particular. I think I was the only evacuee in the school and I was probably considered an outsider in this country town. I guess that living with my teacher would not have helped my classmates to accept me!

The flying bomb attacks at home had lessened towards the end of the year and it was decided that I should return home at the end of the Christmas term. It was thought these raids were coming to an end and it was considered safe to return to Kenton. Perhaps it was inconvenient for me to stay longer, as Miss Rowe's niece would be home for the Christmas holidays. Occasional mysterious "gas main" explosions had occurred in September and at first it was not generally understood that another kind of air attack - rockets - had started, but in my safe country home I knew little of these V2 rockets.

So, just before the end of term, a case containing my clothes was sent off by rail, 'luggage in advance' and addressed to my home in Kenton. As soon as the Christmas holiday began I packed my few remaining possessions into the saddlebag of my bike, together with my School Report and the three scarves I had woven for Christmas presents. Early on the Sunday morning immediately before Christmas Miss Rowe made me some sandwiches (which she called 'mock crab', but was a mixture of grated cheese with a little mustard) to eat on the journey. I left the bungalow in which I had been so happy, and Miss Rowe and I walked down to Wellington Station and waited on a cold, foggy morning for the London train. It was late arriving. Miss Rowe had checked that its destination was Paddington and when it eventually drew in to the station, a porter stowed my cycle away in the luggage van at the back of the long train. I climbed into a carriage and slammed the heavy door behind me, released the thick leather strap, which enabled me to open the window, and waved 'good-bye' to Miss Rowe. I can still see her in my mind's eye, standing on the platform, as we waved our hands vigorously to each other, while the train steamed out of the station. She had cared for me so well and I remember her with affection, although we were always very formal in our relationship. We never kissed each other goodnight and did not embrace even when I was leaving Wellington.

The train was very crowded. People were standing in the corridors and soldiers were sleeping on the floor, sprawled over any available space, using a kit bag for a pillow on which to rest their heads during the long journey home on Christmas leave. I forced my way unsteadily down the crowded, jolting corridor, carefully stepping over, or around, the men on the floor, before I found a compartment that had a tiny space into which I could squeeze myself. I managed to ease into a bit of a seat between two civilians who moved up a little, then quickly hid their heads again behind their Sunday newspapers. Nobody spoke to anyone, and apart from the rustle of newspaper, there was silence in the compartment. Nearly everybody was smoking or snoozing as I settled down in the nicotine filled, hazy atmosphere while I daydreamed of being at home for Christmas. I had nothing to read and just had to sit there for this daylong journey. I wouldn't dream of going on a long journey nowadays without taking a book to read to while away the time, but one didn't own books in those days. I would certainly choose a non-smoking carriage, but would probably suffer the noise of mobile phones ringing, with the enforced listening to one half of innumerable conversations instead!

The train had begun its journey in Penzance hours earlier and was a 'slow' one, stopping at every station. I could have travelled home on a fast train from Taunton but my father thought it was better for Miss Rowe to be able to see that I was safely settled on a London-bound train, and the express train didn't stop at Wellington Station. (There is no railway station at Wellington now; no trains now rattle through.) Our train often halted between stations too, and we sat silent and cold in the unheated carriage in the middle of nowhere, waiting for the signals to change and allow us to crawl on slowly in the fog. After a while I unwrapped my brown paper bag of sandwiches and rather self-consciously ate them while the train was stranded in yet another deserted spot of misty countryside. Nobody spoke. There was no refreshment bar and certainly no possibility of a drinks trolley passing through the crowded corridors, and none was expected.

It must have been around mid-day when we steamed into Temple Meads Station at Bristol, but it seemed later, as it was so dark and gloomy. I had no watch, so had no real idea of the time. There was a long delay, much banging of doors, unhitching of carriages, sounds of shunting and the venting of steam. Information was announced over the loudspeaker, but I couldn't make out what was being said, until I thought I caught the word 'Crewe'. I strained my ears to catch all the words of the muffled voice of the announcer above the noisy bustle outside, but the information was not clear. I grew worried and plucked up my courage to ask the man sitting next to me if we were going to Paddington. He told me that our carriage and several others were being uncoupled to join the train to Crewe. Only the front half of the train was London-bound. Carriages from another train were being transferred on to it, hence all the delay and noise of shunting and bumping. My bit of the train was headed in a very different direction and would leave very shortly for Crewe.

I was quietly terrified, but to my relief this gentleman was willing to help me. He left his seat and rushed along the platform of this murky, noisy station to retrieve my bicycle from the luggage van at the back of the train. We both then ran to the already uncoupled front half. He hurriedly pushed me into a carriage, before taking my bike to the correct luggage van. I was very grateful for his help, and I hope he got back to his own northern-bound train before it left, and that he still had his seat for the remainder of his journey. We were both very anxious that we might each lose our respective trains.

I worked my way along the slightly less crowded corridor of the London train until I found a seat in yet another smoky compartment, desperately hoping that its destination was Paddington and that my bike was in the luggage van. I still had nothing to do or to read to take my mind off the long journey and its uncertainty. I was still not sure whether I was on the right train. It was only when we drew into a big station some time later, and I managed to hear the word 'Reading' over the loudspeaker from the announcer's distorted voice, that I knew I was heading in the right direction - Paddington, and home. I had travelled between Reading and Paddington earlier in the year and so knew that I really was on the right line.

This nightmare journey ended at last, and it was dusk when the train steamed into Paddington Station. I was so relieved to have arrived safely and felt quite confident about my cycle ride home. As the train emptied, I hung around until I could find a porter who would spare the time to hand my bike down from the luggage van. I wheeled it through the station yard and set off on this last stage of my journey. The fog that had accompanied us from Somerset had lifted but there was very little daylight left. My father had thought that as we had cycled home from Paddington Station after our short holiday in the spring. He had reminded me of the route home when I had talked to him on the telephone before leaving Wellington. He had instructed me to come out of the Station into Praed Street and turn left at the end of this road into the Edgware Road. From there it was a straightforward journey to Colindale, where I would turn left again into the Kingsbury Road, which led directly to the familiar territory of Kenton.

Although I had only travelled this route once, just before D-Day, I was sure I could remember the way home. However, I left Paddington Station via the Goods Yard, and not the main exit on Praed Street. Did I cycle down Praed Street and pedal straight across a deserted, unrecognised Edgware Road, only to turn left at the wrong junction? Or had I got on to another small road as I left the Station from the Goods Yard, turned left into Sussex Gardens and then crossed the Edgware Road on to Marylebone Road? I will never know, but on looking at a Road Atlas, the latter seems probable. The London streets were completely traffic free on this wintry Sunday afternoon in wartime. I had taken a wrong turning at some point and soon realised that I was not on the right road home, but how was I to find the right road? I just cycled on, hoping that I would find the right way. The road didn't seem anything like the one I had cycled along in the summer with my father, and I knew that I had gone wrong somewhere. I had been living in a rural environment for some months and was unfamiliar with big city surroundings.

After a while I passed Baker Street Underground Station, which was a familiar landmark because of our day trips up to the West End on the Metropolitan Line. I recognised the Station, but did not recall passing it when we had cycled along the Edgware Road six months previously. My unease increased, but still I cycled on hoping, that I was going in the right direction and would eventually link up with the Edgware Road, but inwardly sure that I had lost my way. There was nobody around to ask. All the streets were empty and dingy, and nothing was familiar. The buildings were very shabby-looking and the area became increasingly run-down, but still I cycled on. It was nearly dark when I saw a sign saying Old Street Underground Station. I was sure I had never seen or heard of this station before. I knew then that I was completely lost. There was nobody around to ask. I knew that the only thing I could do was to turn round and retrace my route to somewhere I knew - like Baker Street Station.

I began pedalling furiously all the way back along what I can now trace from a London street map is the A501 (City Road, Pentonville Road, Euston Road and Marylebone Road), until I saw the Baker Street Station sign again. I almost felt that I had reached heaven! I hauled my bicycle down the steps, bought a single rail ticket to our local Metropolitan Line station of Northwick Park, carried my bike down a second flight of steps on to the platform and sat waiting impatiently, with beating heart, in an empty train. I longed to be safely home. Gradually one or two other passengers appeared, and at last the guard blew his whistle, waved his flag and I knew the train was about to leave. After a twenty-minute journey I reached my destination. I was so relieved. I still had to lug my bike down a further flight of steps at Northwick Park Station and cycle the familiar mile or two to my home, where my father was anxiously awaiting me, wondering what had happened, and why I was so late in arriving home.

He had been unable to bring me home himself on the Saturday because he was at work. He could not take time off for personal or domestic reasons in those days, especially in a shop on the busiest Saturday in the year. Neither could he meet me on the Sunday, as he felt he had to make his usual pre-Christmas visit to my mother. Hospital visitors were restricted to one-and-a-half hours on Wednesdays and weekend afternoons. It was impossible to get to Shenley Hospital during visiting hours after closing the shop at one o'clock on a Wednesday. He was at work all day on Saturday, so Sunday was the only day he could visit my mother. He knew that the Monday, Christmas Eve, would be very busy and so he couldn't have met me if I had delayed my journey for another day, because his inescapable duties had priority over personal needs; we had both been sure I could cope. I had cycled home from Paddington Station the previous summer. I thought that I could remember the way, which was very direct, as long as I recognised where I should turn left into the Edgware Road. Perhaps my few months spent in the country, along with the deserted streets of London at dusk, the gloomy end of the day and the anxiety I had already had on the journey, all contributed to my big mistake.

I shall never forget that journey as long as I live. I think my father, in his own tiredness, the stress of his visit to my mother and his anxiety about my delayed arrival, was cross with me, and didn't understand the problems I had had. I don't remember whether I even told him what had happened on the train journey. This didn't help to make my homecoming a very joyous one, and for a while I felt reluctant to hand over my hand-woven Christmas presents two days later! However, I had recovered by the time Christmas Day arrived and we had our usual quiet celebrations. This very eventful year of 1944 had contained some very happy times but had ended on rather a low note.

Chapter Nineteen

TERMINATIONS

I returned to Chandos after the Christmas holiday to complete what was left of the final (third) year of my secondary education. Nineteen-forty-five was a year of both international and personal completions. The War in Europe was over in May. My secondary education would finish in July. The first atomic bombs used in warfare were dropped on Hiroshima and Nagasaki in August and brought about the immediate surrender of the Japanese. Hostilities in the Far East ceased and World War 2 finally came to an end. Peace would come at last.

Some girls were only evacuated for a few weeks during the summer holiday and had returned home when the flying bomb raids had lessened, but mysterious 'gas main explosions' began to occur in September. The public suspected that these were a new form of enemy action, and the rumour was soon replaced by official recognition that the South of England was enduring a new kind of air attack. The Germans had perfected the world's first rockets, and these V2s, as they were called, were being fired from their launching pads across the Channel even as the Allied Forces were advancing through Europe. There were no air raid sirens, no warning sounds of the approach of a throbbing engine, but from time to time there was a sudden immense explosion when a rocket fell to the ground, causing much more damage and loss of life than the smaller V1 bombs had done. I had escaped the first few months of this new anxiety, but these unannounced air attacks occurred more frequently during the early months of the New Year. Those of us who returned from our safe evacuation were now experiencing a little of the fear and danger that our friends who remained at home had endured for much longer. I have no clear memories of this period apart from recollections of these occasional sudden, unannounced, frightening explosions.

As I look back I am surprised that I did not appear to have missed my own School during the previous term. It must have been good to be back with my old classmates in our old familiar classroom, although I seem to recall a different feeling in the School environment. There were some new girls in my class and many once familiar faces had gone. There was an unsettled, 'unknowing' feel, an atmosphere that things had changed. As so many were evacuated, perhaps two classes had been combined and some girls had been moved up into my old form from another class? Nothing was explained, questions were not asked, but uncertainty persisted. I have many random memories of the period from my return home from Somerset to the time I left School in July. A lot seemed to happen but events seem disconnected.

I remember the School received a large food parcel from Canada towards the end of the War, and a bag of chocolate-flavoured powder was given to each girl. It was a nutritious blend of dried milk, cocoa and sugar, with the addition of some vitamins, and it must have been our first taste of drinking chocolate. We dipped our fingers in the powder and licked them as we walked home with our gift and thought it was delicious. The remainder was used to make milky chocolate drinks without having to add any of our daily fresh milk allowance.

A few rough girls in the School caused trouble now and again. I was once involved in a bit of a skirmish with a girl who set about me for some reason on my way home one afternoon - or, perhaps, for no reason! She was feared by many of us as she was aggressive, rude and a bully, but nobody wondered why she was so belligerent and defiant, or thought that she might have problems at home. She was just a very naughty girl and we tried to keep out of her way. But on the whole we were a fairly easy class to keep in order - I hope the late Miss Oyston would agree! (She died in 2001. I was privileged to go to her funeral and felt that I represented the pupils she taught in those difficult wartime years so long ago.) We felt our form-mistress's power was 'awesome' and would not dream of cheeking her or causing disruption in her lessons. Classrooms were quiet during lesson times.

We needed to make up for further lost hours of education in the few short months that remained before the end of the School Year. Miss Oyston was our Form Mistress again for this Third Year. According to my final Easter report in 1945 there were now only thirty-six girls in 3A instead of the forty-eight in the previous year. In spite of the recent additions to our class, its actual size had reduced by a quarter. Some girls were still evacuated and at least one girl had moved from the area after her home was bombed. Others who were in the upper age range of our second-year class had apparently left the previous July to go to Commercial College - after barely two years of secondary education. The rest of us settled down to work.

I don't recall talking about our evacuation experiences, or knowing where any other girls in my class had been living during the autumn term. We didn't exchange stories about the homes we had lived in, or the schools we had attended, and seemed to lack any kind of curiosity about each other. I think my friend Joan had not returned to School. I didn't ask those who had not been evacuated how they had fared during the flying bomb and rocket attacks. I think people's personal lives were very private when I was young and experiences were not shared as they are today. Friendships were more remote and 'hands off'; we didn't embrace each other and were far less 'stirred up' or emotionally aroused. Perhaps this was an effect of the War in our developing years, or due to the education system or social structure of that time, but I believe that people generally were less demonstrative in the middle of the last century than they are today, and did not express their feelings or share intimate confidences.

I soon discovered that the Prefects had been appointed from among those girls who had remained at school the previous term and they were well settled into their positions of responsibility. Maybe they chatted a little more about their personal lives in the privacy of the privileged Prefects' Room but I had missed this honour, felt left out and perhaps missed out on the companionship of these friends. The House Captains and most Vice Captains had been chosen too.

Although I was very disappointed that I was not among the select band of prefects, the House Mistress of Brockley House had withheld the Vice Captain's position until I had returned to Chandos and I was given this appointment. I felt very honoured, as I had been a loyal and enthusiastic member of my House, and I received and wore my green badge of office with much pride. The House Captain was another member of my class. Beryl and I knew each other slightly, but we were drawn together at this time through our responsibility for our House, and a close friendship developed. We had similar backgrounds. We were both only children; our fathers were both Managers of men's outfitters' shops and both our families had a lodger in their homes to help to 'make ends meet' in those lean days. Beryl's father worked all day on Saturdays, as did my father, and our fathers both had a half-day holiday every Wednesday afternoon on their early closing day. Her mother worked at a local laundry.

Beryl and her parents were members of the Salvation Army, and we were both involved in our respective churches, so had much in common. Our friendship began through the leadership positions we held in our School House, continued through the rest of our time at Chandos and the next two years at Hendon Technical College. Although our lives then moved in different directions, we have remained in touch throughout our adult lives. I enjoyed many hours in Beryl's home during my early teenage years. We played Monopoly in our school holidays and were sometimes joined in our game by the lodger in Beryl's home. Harry was like a property tycoon when playing Monopoly, and his skill at buying up the expensive 'properties' quite outshone our ability at the game.

Mrs. Warren once gave me a little of the tripe and onion stew she was cooking for the family's evening meal. Perhaps I had stayed at Beryl's house a little longer than I should; her dinner was ready, and I had commented on the tasty smell coming from her kitchen. The small portion I was given so many years ago was my first taste of tripe stew since before my mother had her last severe nervous breakdown. Our housekeeper would certainly not have had anything to do with the stomach of an ox, but this dish reminded me of the days when my mother had been at home and in charge of the kitchen and I have never forgotten this tiny incident in Beryl's home. I can recall eating my mother's tripe and onion stew for my dinner when I was very young, with dumplings and flecks of bright green parsley in the sauce. With the appearance of BSE, anything other than prime cuts of beef has become suspect and I haven't eaten tripe for very many years. It was considered a tasty, nourishing and cheap meal when I was young.

One Saturday afternoon Beryl and I went to the matinee at the local cinema to see Charlie Chaplin in his first serious film, 'The Great Dictator', with his derisive caricature of Adolf Hitler. We also saw 'Great Expectations' and a film about David Livingstone's expeditions to find the source of the Zambezi River and Lake Nyasa. I can recall the rather hazy black and white film showing him struggling through the jungle with his porters, desperately weak and ill, but determined to achieve his aims. I vividly remember the eventual meeting with Henry Stanley of the New York Herald and his greeting to the explorer, 'Dr. Livingstone, I presume'.

Around this time I began to spend some of my Sunday afternoons and evenings with Beryl and her parents at Regent Hall, their Salvation Army Corps in the West End of London. As soon as I could get away from home after our Sunday dinner, I travelled up to Baker Street on the now familiar Met. Line from Northwick Park, then changed trains on to the Bakerloo Line to get to Oxford Street Station, and hurried along to 'The Rink', as the Salvation Army Hall was informally called. The building had been an ice rink in the nineteenth century and was bought by the Salvation Army some time in the l880s and altered for their special use. The Corps still has the same premises, which are now much modernised.

The afternoon Meeting had just finished when I arrived, and Beryl and I, along with the other young people who attended regularly, used to lark about, chasing each other through the various rooms in the building before we had tea. Everyone brought their own food and we all shared tea in an upstairs room in Regent Hall. Then we youngsters followed the Band as they marched through some of the surrounding back streets, where they held an early evening open-air meeting. We gathered in a group in a narrow street, with the tall, old, tenement-like houses on either side. The band played, leading us in the singing of the Salvation Army 'songs'. We all sang heartily, hoping the local inhabitants would be able to hear us. An Officer gave a short talk in a loud, clear voice – no P.A. system, just very strong use of the vocal cords! Then we marched behind the band back to Regent Hall for the evening service. I remember attending an open-air meeting at Speakers' Corner in Hyde Park, where a large crowd gathered around us as some of the group gave testimony to how coming to faith in Christ had dramatically changed their lives.

I enjoyed the evening services and the rousing singing very much. The playing of the well-known Regent Hall Band under the direction of Bandmaster Twitchen and the music of the Songsters - the Salvation Army term for the choir - enthralled me. Their harmonious singing was supplemented by skilful use of the tambourines. I joined in the rousing singing of the lively congregational 'songs', listened attentively to the robust preaching of Major Rich, the Officer in charge of the Corps, and was moved by the appeal for folk to come forward to the 'mercy seat' in front of the platform. It was all so very different from the restrained services and slow hymn singing that I was used to in our tiny wooden church. I think my father was quite concerned that I would soon be donning a Salvationist's bonnet! It was straight to bed when I arrived home late on Sunday evenings and back to school the following day.

Food was in very short supply towards the end of the War, and there were even greater food restrictions in place when I resumed my Domestic Science lessons. My friend Beryl remembers the occasion when we had to make a lamb stew. It consisted mainly of vegetables, with a tiny amount of meat in it. When our Domestic Science session was over, Beryl wrapped newspaper around her covered casserole, put it in a paper carrier bag (no plastic bags in those days) and placed it carefully into the saddlebag of her bicycle, padding it around with more newspaper to try to prevent it from slipping. She cycled home cautiously, hoping to keep the casserole level, only to find when she undid the straps of her saddle-bag, that the glass casserole had moved and the contents were spread all over the inside of the bag. There was no stew for the Warren family dinner that night! Rationing became even more severe after the War was over.

The content of the Hygiene lessons I had at school in Wellington are totally forgotten, although the subject is graded in my end of term Report. Neither have I any memory of Hygiene lessons at Chandos. There is no such subject printed on my report for any of the three years I was attending the school. The only hygiene information we received occurred when the 'Nit Nurse' visited the school to examine our hair, looking for head-lice, and inspected the cleanliness of our hands and fingernails. As we queued up to see the Nurse, our interest in this diversion from our lesson was mixed with some apprehension that we might be handed a letter to our parents concerning foreign residents in our hair. This never happened to me, so I have no idea what the suggested remedy was, but I do remember such letters being discreetly handed out from time to time. I recall no sex education of any kind, or any preparation about our approaching (or already, for some, arrived) puberty.

I remember noticing with curiosity signs of small bumps in obvious places and other little mysterious changes in some of my fellow classmates when we were in the showers after our P.E. lessons. A few girls occasionally brought a note from home that appeared to excuse them from having a shower, but my understanding of any possible reason for this was, to say the least, vague. I was physically a 'late developer' and at the age of nearly fourteen I was not aware of any changes in my own body. Buying myself a bra a year or so later was a great embarrassment! We were given no information at School about menstruation or procreation.

However, some limited education about puberty occurred during that summer, after my fourteenth birthday. I came home from school one day and our housekeeper gave me a large adult medical book to read. She was doing the ironing at the kitchen table and asked me to sit down and read a chapter of the hefty book placed on the table by the side of the pile of ironed clothes. She opened it at a particular page and indicated where I should begin reading. I sat and read, and read, on and on. I had little comprehension of the meaning of the complicated medical terms I came across and only a very uncertain idea and, I believe, some embarrassment, of what it was all about. 'Auntie' asked me if there were any questions I wanted to ask, or if there was anything I didn't understand, but I was too embarrassed to ask her to explain more simply what I had been reading. I had long passed the chapter I had been told to read and must have reached some discourse on bowels, because I came across the word 'stool' once or twice, and really could not understand what a stool had to do with the subject of constipation - I knew the meaning of this word! I asked 'Auntie' what 'stool' meant, as I only knew it to be a three-legged, backless seat. It had seemed to me to be a word I could speak aloud and about which I could ask for an explanation. I don't think my reading provided me with any form of sex education and the 'facts of life' were still an unknown mystery to me.

I felt unable to express my real incomprehension about what I had been reading and was relieved when I was told I could go off to do my piano practice. I had certainly not understood what it was all about, but was later informed by a girl in my class, who told me the basic 'facts of life' in very simple terms. We were peering through a hedge in the park on our way home from school one day, looking furtively at a lady walking along the nearby street who was obviously pregnant. I don't think I had noticed an expectant mum before. Not many child-bearing-age couples were around in wartime; most young men were away in the Forces. I found it difficult to accept this girl's explanation of how babies were made, where they came from and what the 'bump' was. When she told me how it got there and how it got out, I was almost numb with shock and disbelief!

I came to understand a little more through reading the agony aunt's page in some woman's magazine, although I don't know where this came from, as 'Auntie' didn't have a weekly woman's magazine. I may have seen it in my friend Joan's home. I never had the opportunity to talk about feminine matters with anyone, had no idea of what was likely to occur in my own body at any time, and we didn't discuss sex in the playground. I was very surprised when my friend Joan told me her mother was expecting 'an addition to the family' and thought it quite strange when I saw Joan's mother wheeling her new baby in a pram sometime later. The words 'pregnancy' or 'menstruation' were never used and terms for parts of the body not expressed. I had never held a baby or had anything to do with one.

When I began my two years' at Commercial College later in the year I had begun to show some interest in boys. Interest in fashionable apparel to attract boys was another matter however, as clothes were still rationed; styles were very austere and simple. We had no smart or 'trendy' clothes and nothing about girls' attire was designed to appeal either to our vanity or to the opposite sex. The 'Utility' symbol meant practicality and usefulness. There were no mini-skirts, long dresses, sportswear, anoraks, trainers, pretty underwear, casual or designer clothes to make us attractive, or to capture the interest of the opposite sex. Everything was made in cotton, rayon or wool. Nylon was only available to those who were able to obtain used parachute material, or who were old enough to be in the right place to meet American soldiers. Modern synthetic, easy-care fabrics had not been invented. Ironing was a real chore!

Austerity ruled and continued to rule for a number of years, before the 'New Look' with full skirts appeared. Clothes rationing continued until l949, when I was eighteen; for eight years there had been no new fashion in clothes. Our clothes certainly would not attract the boys, but neither did the boys have any smart or stylish clothes that would appeal to us - navy or black 'bomber' jackets were the best they could manage for casual wear, and neither sex paid much attention to what the other wore. Girls who had left school had a little more opportunity to make or improvise smarter clothes and develop innovative and creative ideas. They were now at work and had a little money to spend on themselves.

We schoolgirls wore no make-up; our hair was bobbed, held back with a ribbon tied in a bow on top of our head, plaited, or worn in two bunches secured with ribbons at the nape of the neck. We never expected to have any money for 'pampering' ourselves at the hairdressers, or buying accessories, jewellery and make-up; there were no spare coupons to buy clothes for sports or leisure wear.

The Easter term of l945 came and went so quickly. As the month of May began we knew that the War was at last nearing its end, and on Monday, 7th May, we learned from the wireless that hostilities would officially cease the following day. On Tuesday the 8th May Mr Churchill told the country that the War in Europe was finally over, Germany had unconditionally surrendered. Peace was declared in Europe and the country could celebrate. Mr. Churchill ordered that the next two days were to be a national holiday. Red, white and blue bunting could be bought without coupons for the rest of the month. Patriotism was approved of and we were proud of our country. Many street parties were arranged, bunting was hung up from house to house and Union Jack flags draped from windows, but there was no street party in my rather wide main road, where people tended to 'keep themselves to themselves'. There didn't appear to be the same sense of neighbourliness as in the smaller roads. We didn't have bunting or flags hanging from our windows and I don't recall seeing, certainly never attended, one of these famous street parties.

My father decided that we would go up to London and join in the national celebrations in the Capital. We travelled to Trafalgar Square on a crowded underground train, arriving at the top of the escalator to join the ecstatic crowd in the street, moving *en masse* in a swaying sea around Nelson's Column, filling the entire Square, waving their flags, dancing and cheering continuously. We were part of this excited throng that surged down Whitehall, shouting and singing, holding hands with strangers. We stood on the pavement amongst the cheering, euphoric crowds at the end of this famous street, shouting in unison "We want Winnie", "We want Winnie"; everyone was hoping - and expecting - Mr.Winston Churchill to appear on the balcony of the Ministry of Health building. When he eventually came out and stood before us, waving his cigar and giving us his V-for Victory sign, the crowd roared and cheered. A sailor climbed up a lamppost near me, throwing his uniform hat into the air in exuberant jubilation. The spirit of celebration and the excitement of the crowd were irrepressible and indescribable, so ecstatic and yet so meaningful.

We moved on to the Thames Embankment, irresistibly caught up in the surge of the crowd, where we waited until it grew dark enough for the anticipated firework display to begin on the River. It was a wonderful spectacle, with various set pieces and an abundance of colour erupting from the boats and then cascading down from the sky into the water - a sight I had never seen before - but with none of the frighteningly loud bangs that we hear nowadays during most of November and December. We had all had more than enough loud bangs to last us for the rest of our lives and it was sparkle, joy and colour we needed.

At the end of the fireworks display the crowd streamed on as a huge wave to Buckingham Palace, and my father and I eventually found ourselves standing among this solid mass of humanity that covered the space around the base of the

Victoria Memorial, where the flowerbeds now display their seasonal blooms. There were no neatly laid out flowerbeds in 1945. Suddenly the lights came on in all the rooms of the Palace; the blackout curtains had been taken down and it was an extraordinary sight to see the light streaming out from the windows when every building had been in darkness at night for so many years. Thousands upon thousands of thankful people shouted out, "We want the King; we want the King". Time and time again King George and Queen Elizabeth (the late Queen Mother) appeared on the floodlit balcony together with the two Princesses and everyone roared and cheered even more heartily. I don't know how many hours we spent celebrating in London that night, or at what time we arrived home in the small hours of the morning, but we were part of the throng on this memorable occasion. I shall always remember this experience and am so glad that my father took me up to London on Victory Night.

I had not understood much of the progress of the War and certainly did not appreciate the unspeakable horror and suffering that it brought to countless people. I didn't know anyone who had been killed or injured in the bombing, killed in action in the Forces, or who was a prisoner-of-war. My few relatives were all too old to be called up. Participating in the VE Day celebrations may have helped me to understand a little of the reasons for the elation and general rejoicing of all those who had lived through these six long years of War. Nevertheless I had far greater comprehension of it all after I had grown up, which seems to increase the older I become. How blessed my generation has been to be able to bring up our children without the fear of War, and the fear that they could be called up into the Armed Forces to endure the terror that those only a little older than I had suffered. At the time I knew nothing about the horror and degradation of the concentration camps, or of those who grieved sadly at home over lost loved ones or who were consumed with anxiety about those still fighting and still in prisoner-of-war camps.

But this was a night of celebration, a night never to be forgotten, a night of joy. I didn't give a thought about how my mother had spent the War years in a locked Mental Hospital Ward, probably not understanding what was happening in the world outside, or possibly haunted by the memories of the First World War that had so closely preceded this one. I had more or less forgotten all about her, apart from my half-embarrassed message and subsequent question on each of my father's visits to Shenley Hospital.

We went up to London later on in the year to watch the official Victory Parade, and stood on the pavement as the contingents of the Armed Forces marched by with their bands playing. It was very impressive; I had never seen a big procession before, but my strongest memory is not of this, but of the spontaneous joy of the crowds on the streets immediately after peace was declared.

The War in Europe was over but we would have to wait a few more months before we could say that the Second World War had finally ended. I had left School and was on another cycling holiday with my father in Dorset when the end of the War with Japan was announced. We were staying at another boarding house in a village near Dorchester recommended by the Cyclists' Touring Club's Accommodation booklet. This time we had pre-booked and gone by train from Waterloo to Sherbourne and had a very long and hilly cycle ride to our destination. My father must have been very fit in spite of his slim (skinny?) frame because I had found it very hard going, and my pedalling grew slow and laboured on the seemingly endless incline on the road leading out of Dorchester. I longed for our journey to be over. I was more than pleased when we reached the little village of Winterbourne Abbas, unpacked our saddlebags, eaten a meal and I could go to bed.

Although we were a long way away from the coast, and cycling in the hilly Dorset countryside was quite tough, my father decided that we could manage the ride to Weymouth and have a day by the sea. Having sat on the beach for a while, we were queuing up outside a little cafe on the promenade at lunchtime, when the BBC 1 o'clock news, broadcast from inside the shop, announced that Japan had surrendered. The news was passed quickly from person to person in the queue. It was the l5th August and World War Two was finally over, but the Far East seemed so remote to me and I didn't take in the great importance and significance of this day. We spent the afternoon on the beach and had a swim in the sea before cycling back to Winterbourne Abbas. However, this was a future event and is not really part of this story.

After the national two days' holiday for the VE Celebrations we were back in the classroom. I cannot remember any particular celebration at School, but I feel sure that our Headmistress marked this historic occasion in some way. Recollections of the rest of that summer are somewhat faint and rather muddled. There were some unhappy rumblings at home, although I was not sure what the trouble was all about. Perhaps the strains of the War had taken their toll and with the general euphoria and removal of fear, other anxieties remained and personal tensions were intensified and expressed. My father felt that it would be better for all of us if he and I did our own housekeeping and that 'Auntie' and Rose looked after themselves. They continued to live in our house for some years, as alternative accommodation was difficult to find at the time. The back bedroom now became their bed-sitting room with the addition of some furniture of their own that had been in store. We often ate our breakfast together at the kitchen table in an uncomfortable silence, and there was a certain amount of strain between our two small families that continued for a long time, although a few years after they had moved we all became good friends again.

My father began buying the weekly grocery rations at the long-since disappeared Gapp's grocer's shop in Ealing Broadway. He carefully packed our two eggs (when they were available) into an old collar-box, wedging them in with newspaper, before strapping the box on to the carrier at the back of his bicycle, trusting that they would arrive home unbroken! The rest of our rations were tucked into the panniers attached to either side of the back wheel. Food was very scarce after the War and we were sometimes without one egg each for several weeks. I shopped for our meat ration, the vegetables, bread and other items after school. We had our main meal midday at work or school, but I prepared something for our tea. I also did the washing (rubbing vigorously at my father's shirts with a bar of soap on the scrubbing board) and cleaned the house (probably not very thoroughly). It made life rather complicated and busy for me and I didn't have much time for leisure pursuits - but there were not many leisure pursuits in those days.

My memories of this period are rather vague; everything, both at home and at school, seems so disconnected, or as if it was hanging in the air. As I look back on this period there appears to be a semblance of unreality, but I knew that the rest of the term had to be completed before moving on to Hendon Technical College for my Commercial course. We had inter-House competitions for the first time, which Beryl and I, as House Captain and Vice-Captain, had to organise for Brockley House, with the advice and collaboration of our House Mistress, Mrs. Humphries. How fickle is the memory! I have very little recollection of any of the details of these competitions, which at the time seemed to be so important, and can only remember the Poetry Competition.

Mrs. Humphries wanted me to represent my House, and suggested that I recited Kipling's poem, 'The Fuzzy Wuzzies'. This poem reflected a British soldier's feelings about fighting "wiv' many men across the seas and some of 'em was brave and some was not; the Paythan and the Zulu and Burmese, but the Fuzzy was the finest of the lot." It had to be recited with a Cockney accent to be effective and Mrs. Humphries thought this would provoke special interest from the judges. I memorised it, but feared that this vernacular language would not be approved of or thought appropriate by my teachers (who were to be the judges), and especially by Miss Pike, who was to be among those evaluating the efforts of each House. I didn't appreciate that employing some humour and informal expressive language when reciting this poem would be more distinctive and effective than the one I chose.

My House Mistress knew best but I felt that my 'put on' Cockney accent and the slang expressions in the poem would displease the judges and be frowned upon. I recited Wordsworth's sonnet 'Upon Westminster Bridge' instead, but unsurprisingly, despite my best efforts at eloquent declamation, I did not win the Poetry Competition. The final winner of the House Competitions is now completely forgotten, as are many other events in my last few months at school.

'The Fuzzy Wuzzies' would certainly not be approved of in today's politically correct society. In the days of the British Empire Kipling was applauding the strength and bravery of the African tribal enemy in the Boer War and did not consider it any more demeaning than calling the British foot soldiers 'Tommies'. We were unaware of racial differences at school and rarely came into contact with children of another race, colour or religion. I remember seeing a black girl in the playground at my Primary School, but she was not in my Year. A new girl with the surname 'Kohn' joined our class in about 1938. She may have been one of the Jewish children who escaped from Germany shortly before War broke out. I didn't get to know her at all and remember her as being very quiet; perhaps she didn't speak much English. I can picture a girl with long, dark, wavy hair, named Ruth, who was in my class at Chandos, but only realised years later that she was probably Jewish because of her surname and features. Our much-loved second-year form mistress was also Jewish.

The only girl in my class who may have been thought of as 'different' was a Roman Catholic and we didn't understand why Dorothy was not allowed to remain in the classroom for our Religious Knowledge lessons. Roman Catholics were not allowed to take part in any Protestant religious education or act of worship in those pre-Vatican-2 days, although we studied only small parts of the same Bible and received very uncontroversial teaching. She may have felt 'different' because of this. I don't think she was shunned or bullied or left out by her contemporaries, but it was a very divisive ruling that could have been the cause of isolation and bullying in some areas. It was highly improbable that our R.E. teachers would try to emphasise different doctrines of denominational teaching, and no attempt was made to impart any understanding of different faiths. Although Mrs. Humphries was Jewish, we learned nothing specific about present-day Jewish faith and practice - although inevitably our Old Testament theme dealt with early Jewish history. We were unaware of any significance concerning racial or religious 'differences' and officially imposed unifying policies were unnecessary.

Some rather strange activities occurred during that summer term. For some weeks 'Butter-making' was rife throughout the school, as many girls, including me, poured some of our school milk into old medicine bottles. Whenever we were sitting at our desks without a pen in our hands, and during any spare moments during the day, we shook our small bottle of milk from side to side, until the cream separated from the whey and a lump of 'butter' had formed inside the bottle. This shaking was done surreptitiously during lessons, and I sometimes wonder what the teacher's perception, both literal and mental, must have been as she looked at the pupils in front of her, rhythmically swaying from side to side, with their hands neatly held down beneath their desks. Was some unknown nervous affliction spreading through the school in epidemic form? We certainly were, temporarily, a little crazy. The pastime soon died away; we not only grew weary through jiggling from side to side but we found that the 'butter' was sour, unsalted, and inedible when, and if, we managed to force the lump of 'curds' out of the medicine bottle when we got home.

Someone thought of another rather odd, but innocuous, hobby and we began collecting rose petals from our gardens. We placed the petals in small jars with close-fitting lids, topped them up with water, screwed on the lid and left the mixture to infuse, giving it the odd shake or two from time to time. The resulting foul liquid was supposed to be a rose-scented perfume, which was of course quite unsuitable for use. Indeed, when would we want to wear perfume? We did not contemplate wearing make-up in our school days. Rose had begun to buy a few items of cosmetics with some of her weekly wage packet after she started work. (The lipstick was rather noticeable; maybe it was rather a lurid colour or she put on a little too much.) Her mother was horrified, threw the lipstick into the dustbin and rebuked her daughter, telling her, "Princess Elizabeth and Princess Margaret Rose don't go around with their faces plastered in make-up!" I'm not at all sure how she knew this 'inside information'. There was little media exposure of the Royal Family in those days and what there was would only be seen on the cinema newsreels in black and white, or found in magazines with monochrome pictures. Rose went out and bought some more lipstick when she received her next week's wages!

Our simple games, enthusiasms and pleasures seem so trivial and innocent when they are compared with the interests of similar-aged girls today. As schoolgirls we had not thought of boys (well, most of us); we rarely met them. We knew little (or nothing) about sex. We did not use or even yearn for make-up, (there was little in the shops, nor was lavish pocket money given for any precocious school-girls to waste on lipstick or mascara!); designer clothes or trendy fashions had not been thought of. We wore our school uniform during the week and our best clothes, if we had them, on Sundays. 'Pop' music did not exist as a descriptive word, or as a type of contemporary music appealing especially to youth. The popular songs of the day were not especially geared to a youth culture. Everybody listened to the radio, and the wartime songs were sung or whistled by all ages. Records were not in plentiful supply and those that were for sale revolved at 78rpm and were played on wind-up gramophones. We were not sufficiently affluent to save up for anything special, and there was not much of interest to buy in the shops. Our savings consisted of the sixpence or shilling (5p or 10p) we brought to school each Monday morning, along with our dinner money, to buy one or two National Savings Stamps, which we stuck in our Savings books for the future. This gave the country the use of our 'capital' to help with the war effort; our benefit was the minute interest on our minuscule investment piling up for the future!

Were we deprived? Could it be that we were not exploited, not forced into early maturity, or manipulated by external forces into a particular mode of behaviour or kind of culture, but were allowed to develop naturally and gradually and enjoy our childhood and the process of growing up. I knew of no teenage pregnancies, there were no newspaper articles or TV programmes of violent or dysfunctional families, no pressures from peers, magazines or media to push us into 'relationships' or premature love affairs (although I presume these must have occurred occasionally). I am sure that illicit cigarette smoking occurred in the Boys' School, but I didn't know any girls who smoked in the Girls' School. A few may have had a puff behind the bicycle sheds - my un-named graduate friend in Australia and her fellow-adventurer Joy, perhaps? - or when we were away from School premises. Drug taking had not appeared in suburban society in my youth, so that was not a pressure or temptation for any of us; the drug culture did not exist. Alcohol was also outside our experience and there were no drunken, so-called 'right of passage' orgies at the end of our school lives.

We were not taught about our 'rights', or to be assertive. We knew nothing about feminism. We were probably not particularly confident or prepared to express strong opinions. We were not worldly-wise or acquisitive - there was not much to acquire in war-torn Britain, or for some years afterwards. Even though we did not have much materially, we were content. We were the last generation of an old life-style, where, although many mothers of school-age children were at work during the War, a woman's place was still thought of as in the home, with little expectation of career fulfilment.

Opportunities of further education were very limited; commercial or Technical College was our highest expectation. The possibility of going to University, gaining a degree and having a real choice of career was beyond our wildest dreams because we were only in a Senior and not a County or

Grammar School. But we did not even dream of these advantages. By today's standards our education was very brief, limited - and non-existent in many areas - and even our three years of secondary education had been interrupted by the 'doodle-bugs' and the rockets.

We sat our final year examinations and received our last School Reports in sealed envelopes, which were not opened until they had been put into our parents' hands. School reports and class position were very private and personal and were read by parents only. I had been fourth in position in my first year, dropped to sixth in my second year, but in my last year at school I came top of my A-stream class. I am sure my father was pleased with my progress, but very little was made of my modest success. My position is clearly stated at the head of my final School Report, but my father may not have realised the significance of the fact that his daughter was top of the School. No awards were given, we had no Prize-giving ceremony and no Speech Day occurred.

Chapter Twenty

MOVING ON

Beryl and I had a few days' work experience at the laundry where her mother worked before leaving School. 'Little Laundries Ltd.' was very short of staff and we were 'taken on' temporarily over the Easter holiday weekend. We spent each day holding the four corners of damp, newly-washed sheets, giving them a good shake between us to straighten them out, then folding each sheet into a suitably small, neat square. The sheet was added to the pile of laundry waiting to be taken to the drying machines and then to the ironing press. I fear that we were not very proficient at this menial task, nor were we very dedicated to our work. We didn't hold the corners tightly enough, occasionally lost our grip, got the giggles, and the sheets sometimes fell on to the floor. We were rather light-hearted about our responsibilities, and I fear that although the concrete floor of the laundry was clean, a few customers may have received their laundry back a little dirtier than they had sent it. It was very labour intensive work, very boring, and I am sure I would not have lasted long as a laundry Assistant! I took my next job much more seriously.

I started a Saturday job in my father's shop after my fourteenth birthday. My duty at the shop was to act as a store 'detective'. I didn't have to begin my day's work until 11a.m when the shop began to get busy, which gave me a little time in which to do my Saturday household tasks at home before cycling off to work. I was expected to be on the alert for any possible petty thieves, and to act as a deterrent to shoplifters by my eagle-eyed observance of customers as they looked around the shop while waiting to be served.

I tidied the boxes of socks during slack periods, and folded and re-arranged the trays of ties that were displayed in the showcases beneath the glass counter. I was sometimes approached by a customer if all the assistants were busy and I tried to help them by showing items in which they were interested until a salesman became free, but I was not allowed to make a sale, handle any cash or use the till. If someone wanted to buy a tie, I took pleasure in folding a selection of them one by one over my hand in - I hope - a professional manner, to show how well they would look when knotted around the neck. You don't see this done nowadays! I spent my time standing behind the counter, or walking around the shop, keeping my eyes open for any petty thieves, but at the same time trying to look friendly and approachable.

There was no self-service in clothes' shops at that period. Customers were not expected to look over the goods or select what they wanted without assistance. They came into the shop, were greeted by an Assistant who stood behind the counter and very politely asked what 'Sir' or 'Madam' wanted. A selection of the requested item was produced, and the salesman was attentive and deferential, endeavouring to help the customer to make the appropriate choice. When a purchase was made the Assistant received a small commission. The goods were then wrapped in crisp brown paper that was sharply torn from a large roll at the side of the till and then tied firmly with fine, white string.

Each member of staff had a short coffee and tea break. On Saturdays another chair was squeezed into the little mirror-walled fitting-room or 'cubby-hole' as the staff called it, to enable me to have my morning cup of 'Camp' coffee, or mid-afternoon cup of tea with my father. We boiled the kettle on an electric fire and this small heater also warmed the tiny cubicle. My father and I sat reading the daily paper between us as we had our drink. My eyes frequently lifted from the paper to look in the mirrored walls, where I saw countless repetitions of the scene in seemingly endless reflections from the four glass walls, before the next Assistant tapped on the door before entering to have his short break.

When everyone had finished their drinks it was my job to take the used cups to the nasty old-fashioned sink 'out the back' and wash them up in cold water with no detergent. I dreaded having to use the ancient lavatory adjacent to the yellowed, stained, crazed sink. Standards of hygiene for the staff were very basic and 'out the back' was in strong contrast to the spotless shop with its polished floors, shiny glass countertops and gleaming mirrored walls.

It was difficult to get adequate and suitable staff during, and for some time after, the War. Unless he was in a reserved occupation or had a physical disability, any young man over the age of eighteen was called up into the Forces. Compulsory National Service did not end until 1953. I remember one of the shop assistants suffered from asthma and my father's 'First Man' had failed his 'Call Up' medical examination because he had flat feet. My father often wondered how this tall, strapping young man was able to stand all day in the shop and yet was considered unfit for National Service. I remember Mr. Wilmot very well and he was very reliable, trustworthy and personable. He was 'First Man' (Assistant Manager) and he and my father only ever referred to each other as Wilmot and Mr. Brook. Apart from the Manager, the rest of the staff were referred to by their surname alone. No first names were used at work, although I knew Mr. Wilmot's Christian name was Dennis from the greeting on the Christmas card my father sent each year after he retired.

He often had a very brief break period himself because he was worried about leaving the shop inadequately supervised while he was shut away from them in the corner 'cubby hole'. He was often very short of staff, and this concerned him greatly during his lunch hour or tea breaks, when insufficient responsible salesmen manned the shop in his absence. Some of the assistants were very inexperienced, and not all were competent or trustworthy. Although female assistants were not previously considered appropriate in a menswear shop, he employed a lady on his staff at one time. Mrs. Goodenough was more than good enough and was a very trustworthy, dependable, affable and efficient lady. I only managed to get my Saturday job with Meakers because my father was in urgent need of additional help. I enjoyed working there, felt very responsible, and I was interested in observing the customers, appearing friendly towards them, or to notice any unusual mannerisms, but it was not a particularly stimulating day's work and when we were not busy the hours dragged by.

The shop door was shut promptly at closing time to prevent any more of the public from entering. Last minute customers were not encouraged, but if they were in the shop they were dealt with politely. Secretly the staff were longing for them to leave, and when the customer had completed his purchase the shop door was quickly unlocked and opened just sufficiently to allow him to leave, and then as rapidly closed again, with the catch put down on the lock, to prevent anyone else from slipping in. Only after the last customer had gone could my father begin to count the day's takings in coins and pound notes. It was unusual to see a five-pound note. Customers paid for their purchases in cash; cheques were rarely handled and of course credit cards had not yet appeared.

Unless the cash balanced with the total recorded by the old-fashioned till roll, the Manager and his 'First Man' were unable to go home. If any discrepancy occurred, it had to be made up by my father, but this very rarely happened. Occasionally he had to check and recheck the total – no calculator to help him - and only when the cash balanced with the till roll was the money placed into a large leather bag, the Night Wallet. This was securely clasped and locked, then taken by my father, accompanied by his 'First Man', to the Night Safe set in the wall of the nearby Midland Bank on the corner of shabby-looking Orchard Street - now pedestrianised and looking very trendy with its pavement cafes and specialist shops.

Only then could we begin our journey home, usually on our bicycles. It was such an awkward journey by public transport, with consequent queuing for buses and waiting for trains that my father preferred to cycle, unless the weather was very wet or icy. He was also able to save the money that would have been spent on fares and put it towards our household expenses. It seemed a long day, even though I had not arrived until mid- morning, and it was tiring standing around all day long in artificial light with nothing specific to do except be watchful. I felt separated from the busy world passing by outside in the daylight. However, I was pleased to receive my small wage for my day's work (I forget how much I earned) that gave me a little money to spend as I was growing up, although I don't remember anything specific, or even any clothes that I bought for myself until I had a full time job.

During the short daylight hours in winter, or if business had been slack, I was sometimes allowed to leave work before closing time. It was not a pleasant cycle ride, with a long pull up Hanger Lane Hill from Ealing Common to the Western Avenue/North Circular Road intersection. This is now one of the most congested areas around North London, and it would be a brave person who would contemplate cycling around it today! It was very different in the l940s, with few cars and no heavy lorries. I cycled on through the light industrial areas and miserable shops around Alperton (which look little different today), up and down the little hills and longer inclines that are not apparent when in a car, until I reached' home.

it is difficult to recognise the present Ealing Broadway shops from how they looked years ago, when the Broadway was lined with 'classy' shops like Meakers, Abernethy's the tailor's shop, Gapps the grocer's and Burtons. Sanders and Sayers were both family-run Department Stores - all quite different and more individual than today's shops, with fine-looking shop fronts. Zeeta's was a very nice café where I remember my mother buying me a 'Buzz Bar' chocolate biscuit to nibble while she had a pot of tea when I was very small.

Senior School days would soon come to an end. Our formal education had been extremely limited, but we had learned some basic principles, understood the concept of loyalty and hard work, knew right from wrong, had a working knowledge of the English language to give us a start in life and could spell! We were numerate and literate. We had developed principles of honesty and unselfishness and perhaps learned, even through our wartime deprivations, many valuable lessons for life. I had lived through so many varied experiences during those three eventful years. Perhaps my real 'secondary' education was still to come; the 'primary' - and the really important - aspects had already been absorbed.

Miss Pike had often made our Friday afternoon Assemblies special and important. Sometimes she invited an outside speaker to address us and occasionally a celebrity came to the School, but I can only remember the name of Miss Dimbleby, the Head Librarian at Kenton Library, who came and spoke one Friday afternoon. She was Head Librarian when the Library opened when I was a little girl, and I admired this tall lady with fair, and what appeared to be naturally curly hair, spectacles, and a friendly smile whenever she date-stamped my Library books. She occasionally had to quietly quell over-loud conversation in the Children's Library in her soft-tones voice. Perhaps she was a member of the famous Dimbleby family?

House Marks were added up for each of the four Houses before our final Assembly at the end of the summer term. Each class filed into the School Hall on that Friday afternoon at the end of July and everyone stood until Miss Pike entered, preceded by the Head Girl carrying the School Shield. After a few introductory comments the entire School sang the 'leavers' hymn, which also had a line in it referring to 'those returning', after which everyone, with the exception of the Teachers and the Prefects who had chairs, sat cross-legged on the floor.

There was always an air of anticipation as the name of the winning House was announced. The appropriate coloured ribbon - red, green, blue or white - was tied around the School Shield with an impressive bow at the front. During the school holidays the winner's name and the year would be engraved on a small shield - for posterity - and fixed to the large one. (No-one is bothered about School Houses with shields of achievement now!) All our End of Year Assemblies seemed significant and the one at the end of my School career was even more important to me. Although I was Vice Captain of Brockley House in my Third and last Year, I cannot remember which House was the winner at the end of the Summer Term in 1945. I can only assume that it was not Brockley House!

After a little homily from Miss Pike the entire School joined with enthusiasm in singing the School Hymn. It seemed particularly meaningful to those who were leaving. The words were very emotive, urging us to despise selfish ambition, to speak the truth, to think the best of those around us, to work for worldwide truthfulness, to defend the right and support the weak; praying that God would grant that we would always keep these vows we made in our song. The words and music had been especially composed when the School first opened. I knew the words by heart and sang this hymn with passion on my last day at School and with tears in my eyes. The sentiments expressed in our School Hymn summarised the ethos that Miss Pike had tried to instil in us, and I am sure that many have been influenced throughout their lives through singing this song at the end of term, and particularly at the end of their school career.

Our final Assembly closed with staff and pupils saying our School Prayer, which members of the Staff had compiled when the School first opened in 1939. Each teacher had contributed her own particular thought to the Prayer, in which we thanked God for the architects and workmen who built the School and for those who maintained it. We prayed that we would always give each other unselfish assistance and cheerful loyalty and that the friendships formed at School would be lasting and sincere. As members of Chandos we were to build a School of fine tradition for those who came after us. We asked for a sense of duty and strength of will to carry out these aims, and prayed that as we left we might take with us happy memories. I certainly left my School with good memories that have remained with me over the years. Some of my old classmates have a Reunion each year we all consider that the values and principles we absorbed in our schooldays have affected our lives for good and look back on our 'Senior School' education with affection and gratitude.

This Assembly was very moving, and after singing the School Vesper and we were dismissed for the last time. I was reluctant to leave the building. I wandered around the School getting friends and staff to sign my autograph book and saying good-bye to some of my teachers. I joined a little group of girls standing around Miss Oyston on the main staircase. She had been my Form Mistress for two of my three years and she was much respected. Although she was not to be trifled with, and was a strict disciplinarian, I was very fond of her. I felt very emotional at the thought of saying 'goodbye' to her, but was surprised when she noticed me among the group of girls. Miss Oyston put her arms around me and gave me a hug, patting me on the shoulder and saying "Oh, Sheila, don't cry!" This was a uniquely demonstrative action in my experience. However, I began to realise that I was now a 'leaver' and no longer part of the School.

Most of the girls were gradually dispersing and many were on their way home. I began to understand that it really was the end of term; the holidays had started. I had indeed left School, and the near-empty building began to feel as if I was about to move out of an old home to a new house and garden. I didn't belong in the old one any more. It was time for me to move on.

Printed in the United Kingdom
by Lightning Source UK Ltd.
120312UK00001B/2